loving
life

loving life

Steve Ford

Dedicated to all of the healthcare professionals around the world who make the impossible, possible.

Contents

Introduction

Whilst in lockdown during the year of Covid, in France, the artist David Hockney said something that has resonated within my soul.

> The **cause of death is birth**. The only real things in life are food and love in that order; just like our little dog Ruby. I really believe this and the source of art is love. I love life.

I love life, and it is probably fair to say that the vast majority of us feel exactly the same way.

Where and how we live is often down to us, and when opportunities present themselves to make changes there is often a dilemma and soul-searching, for fear of the unknown.

Life, however, has a way of forcing change upon us that we didn't see coming... Cancer.

Before I continue, I need to emphasise that this is a positive story and I hope an uplifting one, that as an author I feel compelled to write and share. This time it is personal, very personal and close to my heart, as it centres on my partner and lays bare the impact not just to her, as she embarked on a journey, but on me as a partner, her family and all of those whose hearts she touched.

Amber coped in a way that I did not expect and, as a result, has for me, as a retired airline pilot obsessed with maintaining control, been humbling. The real heroes are all around us, in the street, at work, at play and in our community.

Amber is a cancer survivor and the intention, over the course of the chapters ahead, is to share with you a partner's perspective; what worked, what didn't, the lows and the highs of life with cancer as an unwelcome breast guest.

There is a lot of material out there, and quite rightly so, providing guidance for the patients.

But I found that for partners and loved ones it is a little bit more difficult to get to grips with the impact during and post-treatment in terms of, what do I do? How do I cope and where do I start?

Cancer impacts all genders. It has no boundaries.

The view of a partner, written as honestly and as candidly as I can, hopefully, will be of benefit to those of you finding yourself in fear of the unknown.

Fears can be conquered... believe me.

01 Giving Back

We all harbour good intentions and giving back is something we often try to do. Sometimes we do this in a small way and sometimes, in a big way.

When my partner was diagnosed with breast cancer, I knew it was life changing for her, but I did not realise at the time how significant an impact it would have on those of us around her.

As unusual as it seems, the only way I can start writing this book is by starting at the end.

The experience of the last two years has taught me a lot, not just about myself, but my partner who has undergone the challenges of being diagnosed at a relatively young age, forty-two. It should always be remembered though that cancer knows no limits and can impact anyone at anytime, regardless of age.

I am, as mentioned in the introduction, a retired airline pilot and, whilst having written and published two aviation-related books, the inspiration for this book is Amber, the true heroine.

Or so I thought as, over the last few years, it is the scientists, the oncologists, consultants, nurses and healthcare professionals that are the true unsung heroes.

Our story is not too dissimilar to many; we have both been married before and have been together, to date, because we want to be.

That's a pretty good starting point in our humble opinion.

We have an age difference of nineteen years and whilst Amber never had a problem with it when we met, it certainly played on my mind, the simple reason being that I did not want her, to be blunt, to be burdened with an old, bolshie aviator in the future, trying to decide which care home to shove him into!

My daughter has always said, "It's OK, Dad, it will be a shitty care home so we can save the money!"

Charming.

Joking apart, it never entered my head, or Amber's for that matter, that she would need support and care from not just me, as a partner, but family and friends, overseen by healthcare professionals, to make damn sure she outlived me.

I had retired from long-haul flying before the pandemic hit in 2020, so like everyone else I had asked myself, "What the hell is this all about?"

We lived in the south-east of England and decided, as part of the lockdown "re-evaluation of life" process so many went through, to move.

Whilst family and friends remained in the south, we felt that the West Midlands, which are in the heart of England, in the literal sense, would serve us well.

One of Amber's twin boys was working at Coventry Airport as an aircraft mechanic, and the other was at Farnborough serving an aircraft apprenticeship working on business jets. I know what you are thinking... yes, I am a bad influence!

My son, by his own admission, is a "boffin", as he is a scientist working for a Dutch research institute in the field of molecular biology.

My daughter intersperses backpacking around Southeast Asia with working full-time in software development for various NHS (National Health Service in the UK) Trusts.

In fact, when the pandemic hit she was in a remote part of Cambodia when I managed to connect with her and have the fatherly "You better scoot back pronto" conversation that parents all over the world were probably having at the same time.

South Warwickshire is an area I knew reasonably well and, following a couple of visits staying in hotels in between lockdowns, we decided this is where we wanted to move.

Royal Leamington Spa sits astride the River Leam and this, in turn, runs into the River Avon. Across the River Avon is Warwick, a medieval town complete with castle, Tudor houses and tourists.

To the west is Stratford-upon-Avon, the birthplace of William Shakespeare, attracting even more tourists.

Leamington Spa, however, is in our humble opinion the jewel in the crown for it was developed by the Victorians as a spa town. The result being that the streets are wide to accommodate a coach and six horses, flanked by Georgian-style mansions and villas. There are more parks than a dog walker could ever wish for and more coffee shops than anyone with a good book could dream about.

In February 2021, we moved to Leamington Spa and I started a small aviation consultancy business at Coventry Airport.

We already had good friends in Leamington Spa and soon found that we quickly had more. There is open warmth and hospitality in the Midlands, in fact, and, not intentionally wishing to offend Londoners, exists anywhere outside of the influence of London.

It is true of any big city – New York, LA – their pace of life and high-density populations as urban areas generate their own tension; something we wanted to avoid.

Even though we are just south of Birmingham, which is no village retreat, the pace of life in Warwickshire was just what we wanted. As time went by, we found that our relationship with the town just grew, as we kept discovering more little gems. Whether it is theatre, live music or good restaurants, it's all here.

Life was good until the day the panic button was well and truly hit, the year we had moved to a different part of the country.

Amber was diagnosed with breast cancer on October 22nd 2021.

What has transpired since has been truly inspirational, when I look at the woman that day to the woman I see before me today.

Amber suffered before her diagnosis from anxiety, which she will readily admit, a phobia of hospitals and absolutely no interest whatsoever in working in the medical profession.

For someone who initially adopted the hide under a rock approach to the problem, to be donning the blue tunic of a clinical support worker, off this morning to work in a hospital, has been nothing short of a miracle.

Realising, as we both did, that people are dealing with cancer day in, day out and gaining the support of other patients, it drove her to wanting to give something back.

During her treatment, she engaged with people through social media and it helped her cope. Some people choose to remain private, but Amber chose to face up to her fears and face them head-on. She felt she had to.

Her story is told in her own words on her social media feed[1].

Her own words regarding giving back cannot be paraphrased and should be included in this book from the very beginning. As a partner, I now want to do the same and, as an author, share with you the world of cancer as I witnessed it, day in, day out. It is something I hope that will help all the families and friends of those who surround a loved one.

But first, over to Amber from her post in the spring of 2023:

> *Pre cancer I had a massive hospital phobia. Really hugely massively massive. I didn't know how I was going to cope with all of the hospital appointments. But here I am with the appointments now tailing off, and me feeling a bit sad that soon I will not see any of the amazing nurses ever again.*

---

1. https://www.instagram.com/unwelcome_breast_guest/

As of today, that's all changed. I'm stepping into the world of nursing. Starting off as a Clinical Support Worker within the chemo suite with the goal of becoming a chemo nurse in a few years.

It's an exciting and scary time, but I know it will be so rewarding.

I am so looking forward to being part of our amazing, wonderful NHS.

02 Panic Button

What had I done?

I must have done something.

For weeks, I picked up on an air of angst from Amber and I could not for the life of me work out what I had done.

Left the toilet seat up? No.

Been grumpy? OK, occasionally, I didn't think excessively, though, for someone who had retired from a life of world travel, hotels and the warmth of the sun in late autumn in the Caribbean.

My daughter had already given me the thumbs up when I had asked her what it was like having me around more and not be travelling around the planet in a state of constant jet lag.

She had replied, "It's great, Dad... You're not so much of an arse." You can see already, my daughter keeps me in check.

What had I done?

The weekend was OK, as far as weekends go, and one thing we have never had and never do in our relationship is bicker or argue. If something needs sorting, we just get on and sort it out. But there was something not right and I couldn't put my finger on it.

What I could sense, however, was that Amber wasn't happy with something and I was beginning to worry.

I knew there had been a lot of pressures on her, on us, on everyone with the pandemic and lockdowns; uncertainties, communal stress about where the hell were you going to get toilet paper from if it carried on much longer.

Dawn was later and later each day as autumn started to envelop the northern hemisphere and, in silence, we awoke on the Monday morning.

As I got dressed, and as Amber sorted herself out, I tried gently to get to the bottom of what was eating her up. As I did so, she withdrew more and more, and I suddenly had this horrible pit of the stomach feeling... she didn't agree with my daughter, she thought I was a complete arse!

She quickly reassured me it was nothing of the sort and fell straight back into what I can only describe as a state of depression.

So, I tried to reassure her that we were OK, safe with a roof over our heads, financially secure and surrounded by people that cared.

"And... That the most important thing we've got is our health."

Well that did it!

She burst into tears and, sobbing in my arms, said... "I've got a lump in my breast and I'm scared... I don't know what to do!"

I felt sick to my stomach but, at the same time, in a bizarre way, relief... Now I understood what was going on and, most importantly, now I could help. Something she was readily prepared to let me do.

How someone shares their concerns, when and to whom, is always going to be different. It's too easy to criticise and say, oh, for goodness' sake, you should have done this or you should have done that! Something that is easy to say from the outside looking in. We are all different, and some people march themselves off to the doctor's and some people need support to get there, mentally and physically. Amber needed support.

She was in such a state of shock that it took a while to coax from her gently the facts that I needed.

How long had the lump been there...? Over a month that she had been aware of, but as she explained, often what feels like a lump could be a blockage or associated with a menstrual cycle and some medical practitioners advocate waiting a month.

It's natural to ignore things and see if things improve on their own.

The problem I now faced was she had convinced herself that she only had twenty-four hours to live and who was going to look after the boys and the cat... knowing full well the cat was not impressed with me one little bit as a caregiver.

This is where my training kicked in and I literally pushed emotion to one side.

On an aeroplane, in the flight deck, there is no panic button.

They may well have one down the back, amongst the passengers, but for those at the front we have to deal with it, whatever "it" is.

It was time to take control of the clock, and any pilots out there reading this will know exactly what I am talking about, for the most important instrument in an aeroplane amongst all of the bells and whistles is the clock.

When something happens in an aircraft, there is a split second when you punch through the startle factor and determine; is what's just happened or happening going to kill me in five seconds, five minutes or five hours?

You then react accordingly.

In the first five seconds, you initiate the memory/recall items that will move you into a position where you now have five minutes. Then working through checklists and manuals, whilst aviating, navigating and communicating, you come up with a plan. Once the situation is under control, you have time with which to conclude the journey, safely.

"Let's get you a doctor's appointment straight away" was my immediate recall item, and Amber asked if I could arrange it as, by this time, she was literally curled up in a ball on the bed.

I could see that her anxiety and fear had become debilitating, to a point where she could not function.

I managed to get through eventually to a receptionist at the local surgery, and she took on board my concerns and arranged for a phone consultation that afternoon but needed me to put Amber on the phone for her consent, which, amongst her tears and shaking, she was able to do.

Calming down, she started to rest and immediately I knew we had punched through the first part and at least now a doctor's call was planned that afternoon.

Whilst Amber rested, I phoned one of our good friends who is a nurse. At first, I had to leave a message, but it was not long before she called back and I explained to her what was going on. She immediately volunteered to call around later that day as she was administering Covid jabs close by.

The reality was, I had now transferred all of my angst and concerns to people that could provide guidance. I was out of my depth and certainly not equipped to move forwards on my own. I needed help.

After the doctor's phone consultation that afternoon, an appointment at the surgery was scheduled for the next morning.

Our guardian angel, Beq (pronounced Bex) came around and spoke to Amber whilst I shuttled tea back and forwards. The soothing support from Beq was what was needed, as Amber's phobias were very real and in overdrive. It had not been long since Amber and her sister had been in hospital with their stepfather when he passed away; something that had not only traumatised her, but had cemented her fears, as he had lost his fight with cancer in front of them.

The next day we drove to the doctors, and I had to let her go in on her own due to Covid restrictions.

Part of me wanted to wrap my arms around her and start doing everything for her. Not Amber. She is a tough, independent woman and I knew she had to be given the space to come to terms (as did I) with what the hell was happening.

This carried across to everything, including when, how and what she told family and friends. She was now in charge of the clock.

That Tuesday evening was a difficult one, as the doctor had felt that a full referral to the hospital was required and would make arrangements accordingly.

I knew that the NHS was completely logjammed, as we lurched from Covid outbreak to outbreak. There were waiting lists for everything, and I didn't expect it would be quick enough to obtain a referral.

Early diagnosis is key and we hear it repeated again and again with cancer, something Beq had stressed the night before. It's the waiting that is the worst bit; waiting for appointments, waiting for diagnosis and, if it is cancer, waiting for a plan to lead to treatment.

The day treatment starts is the day a cancer patient is on track.

I could see that the anxiety and fear were imbedded in Amber, so I then proposed that I look and see what options there were to go private and get her seen to straight away for an examination and biopsies, something the doctor had stated as being required.

She agreed and, as a result, I contacted one of the many online cancer-screening services[2] in the UK, and the guy I spoke to was absolutely fantastic, professional, calm and reassuring; exactly what I needed.

Throughout this book, where appropriate, I will provide links and sources of reference material. It must be emphasised that in no way is this meant to be a product or a service endorsement. If it helps, it helps.

The other obvious caveat is the fact that we are in the UK. Therefore, wherever you are on the planet, your country and your region will have different source information, something that should be sought based on your needs and requirements.

I know private is not for everyone and a lot of people simply cannot afford to go down this route, but it was something at that moment in time that was right for Amber.

The doctor came back with an NHS appointment at Warwick Hospital for two weeks' time, whereas

---

2.   https://www.check4cancer.com/

private was available at Sutton Coldfield, to the east of Birmingham, that Friday.

The thing that people often don't know (and I certainly didn't until it was explained to us) is that you can step in and out of private. In other words, whilst the appointment for mammograms, ultrasounds and biopsies was at Sutton Coldfield, and we would have to pay for it, Amber could then go back into the NHS for diagnosis and, if required, treatment. Something she ended up doing.

But what it did achieve, getting an early assessment, was that it shifted the timeline in her favour, it brought forwards everything, and this was priceless.

I have to be careful not to paint a rosy picture about how easy it was. It wasn't. It can officially be classified as a "shitshow". It probably has to go down as one of the worst weeks ever.

Amber curled up in a ball all week and shed a lot of tears, as she had convinced herself, based on the doctor's demeanour, that this wasn't a fatty lump or blocked gland.

Conversations were starting to take place with family members all of which were initiated by Amber and the level of stress rose exponentially.

On the Friday, I drove Amber to Sutton Coldfield, as it is not the easiest of places to get to when you are freaking out with fear, and she gladly accepted my offer to drive.

It was cold and wet, with a typical October lashing of horizontal rain, and when we arrived in the car park, I gave her a hug before she went in. I had to sit in the car as Covid restrictions were still in place and nobody, other than patients, was allowed into the hospital.

Amber's dad phoned me, and I assured him she was coping and that no doubt she would speak to him that evening when we got home. He was worried, I was worried; we were all worried.

As the hours went by, I tried to sleep after reclining the car seat and I felt awful, putting it down to mental exhaustion.

The light was fading as the afternoon wore on, and I could see in the distance someone working their way through the car park tapping on windows. Windows would wind down and it soon became apparent that it was a nurse asking something, as she continued to approach more vehicles.

I was parked towards the back of the car park, and I started to feel sick as I realised she was looking for someone. No not me, please.

As I wound down the window, she said, "Are you Steve? Here with Amber?"

My heart sank.

I walked into the hospital lobby and duly put on a fresh mask and sanitised my hands. I followed the nurse through to a room that looked like a reception area. Off this main room were rooms with machines and another nurse appeared introducing herself as Moira (not her real name out of respect for privacy).

"Amber's just having her biopsies and, when they are done, she will be back and I can explain a few things."

When Amber returned she looked as cool as a cucumber, but all I could do was crumble.

Moira then proceeded to explain to Amber and I what the next step was, and it became pretty clear pretty quickly that what they had seen on the examination and mammogram made them suspect that it was a cancerous tumour, close to her chest wall, and a big one at that.

I felt helpless.

A lot of what was being said just washed over me, and it was only later in the car driving home that I started to file it away into any semblance of order.

What I do remember was hearing that treatment would be a journey of approximately a year if the biopsies confirmed what they suspected.

Armed with leaflets, we headed home and knew that all we could do was wait; wait for the call to go back in and for Amber to receive the diagnosis.

The weekend was surreal, as we were both exhausted and I just could not think straight.

Amber started to struggle with the "telling" family and quite rightly decided that, until the diagnosis, she would limit who she spoke to. There was nothing to tell.

Two days later, feeling like I was being torn apart, I tested positive for Covid. Just what we needed; when it rains, it pours.

I slunk off to the spare room, but it was too late; Amber came down with it and tested positive as well.

We were waiting for the diagnosis but, because we were infected with Covid, no way could the hospital have us anywhere near them.

They arranged a Microsoft Teams call and, on the 22nd October, we sat on the sofa and clicked "*Join the meeting*".

03 Diagnosis

Sat on the sofa, we listened to the diagnosis.

A lot was said, as we stared at the tablet screen, and most of it went in one ear and out the other.

The one thing I do remember is the confidence with which Amber was told and the clarity on what the next sequence of events could possibly be, once the diagnosis was forwarded to the doctor and consultant surgeon.

Different cancers require different approaches... that much was clearly evident based on our limited knowledge to date.

Some tumours are approached from the get-go with chemotherapy, some involve what's called a lumpectomy, which, as the name implies, just involves immediate surgery to remove the lump. If the margins of the removed tumour are completely clear and post-surgery analysis (very important) supports it, that's it! No chemotherapy, any radiotherapy or continuation treatment other than follow-up scans.

However... do not take the above statement as complete... it is not! There are many subtypes of every cancer and treatment can involve chemotherapy and radiotherapy even if there are clear margins. Each and every diagnosis and treatment is tailored to the individual.

Other plans require a mastectomy straight away.

Amber was recommended to consider the latter, as the size and proximity of the tumour to her chest wall meant there were no other options. This, coupled with confirmation by the biopsy that her lymph nodes in her left arm were involved, would require simultaneous surgery to remove these nodes as well.

It all sounds confusing but, in reality, it all had logic to it, as each stage then determined the treatment plan to follow.

Once the "thing", as Amber called it, was physically removed, the lab could then determine from analysis how extensive it was and from the lymph nodes determine if they were all involved.

So what was the diagnosis?

We learned that the cancer was hormone-positive (meaning it's fed by hormones) and HER2-negative.

We had no idea or understanding of the HER2 part, but in simple terms, from what we could gather, HER2-negative suggested that it was likely to grow more slowly and therefore was less likely to reoccur.

Further testing proved it actually to be HER2-positive.

> *HER2-positive breast cancer is a breast cancer that tests positive for a protein called human epidermal growth factor receptor 2 (HER2). This protein promotes the growth of cancer cells[3].*

It was also grade 3. Grade 1 being cancer cells that look like normal cells and grade 3 apparently are abnormal cells that could grow and spread more aggressively.

The grading system confused me. It still does.

---

3. https://www.mayoclinic.org/breast-cancer/expert-answers/faq-20058066

We often hear of stage 4 cancer as being the worst in terms of survivability, but it must be emphasised that people do and continue to survive. There was no mention of stages, just grades[4].

We were full of Covid, and Amber was at peak infection in terms of her strength and generally feeling crap.

We both felt numb after the call and spent the weekend concentrating on recovering from Covid, knowing that the treatment system was kicking in and further consultations would soon be booked, in order to schedule surgery.

On the Monday, it hit Amber and she readily admits she had a meltdown so called Moira, the breast cancer nurse at Sutton Coldfield. Once again, she was amazing. She answered all of Amber's questions honestly and with positivity. She reassured her that she had a lot to be positive about regarding her diagnosis. Providing it hadn't spread beyond her lymph nodes, it was totally treatable and even if it had spread, then because of the type of cancer she had, it would still be very manageable.

4. https://www.nhs.uk/common-health-questions/operations-tests-and-procedures/what-do-cancer-stages-and-grades-mean/#:~:text=stage 3 %E2%80%93 the cancer is,part of the immune system)

The big thing that she picked up on during the conversation was that the nurse was using the word "future" a lot. So Amber tentatively asked whether she still had a "future" if her cancer had spread. Without hesitating, Moira said, "ABSOLUTELY."

Breast cancer is seen by society as affecting women.

Unfortunately, cancer does not differentiate between genders and whilst statistically lower in men, it can develop.

The big problem being that whilst increased awareness and visibility to symptoms and treatment are promulgated in the media for women, it is rarely reflected in the male world.

The second problem is one of early diagnosis, with men not being educated on what to look for and the simple fact that it is a risk that is simply overlooked.

A recent British TV soap did run a storyline where a lead male character did develop breast cancer.

There is a lot of information out there and, witnessing what Amber was going through, it encouraged me to seek out more facts[5]. Something

5. https://www.bcrf.org/blog/male-breast-cancer-statistics-research/

I would certainly encourage any of you to do.

I have to add in a disclaimer here. I am not a doctor; I have no medical knowledge whatsoever other than my experience as part of aircrew medical training practising CPR.

When reading this, for goodness' sake, please take it for what it is and do not necessarily read across from it to your situation or that of a loved one's. A diagnosis is individual, but without it, you cannot move forwards.

It was now time for Amber to take the first steps towards treatment.

04 Hope

Following the first few weeks, Amber managed to pull some hope from her initial shock.

Step by step.

It was a pivotal point as, up until then, her anxiety and hospital phobia had been the overriding factors that dominated every second of the day, and she was wiped out.

In her own words, she summed it up as follows:

'Hope' became my new favourite word.

When I first went to the doctors, we had hoped that I would be told it was nothing to worry about.

When an urgent referral was made for me to go to the breast clinic, we hoped that a quick ultrasound would be enough to suggest that I had nothing to worry about.

Despite being informed that it was most likely breast cancer, we still hoped that the biopsy results would show that the lump was anything other than cancer.

I noticed a change in her demeanour; yes, there was still a very frightened woman, but there was also a spark of determination and sheer bloody-mindedness to get through this and come out the other side as one of the millions of other cancer survivors out there.

It happened without my input whatsoever and only happened when she was ready. I was not the one diagnosed with cancer; coming to grips with it and managing the clock were her call.

What happened next surprised me. I did not see it coming, and I think it is fair to say that none of our family and friends did either.

She had started to search out information and build up a better understanding about this new world.

One book that became the source of her desire to fight back was *Glittering a Turd: How surviving the unsurvivable taught me to live* by Kris Hallenga.

As a result, Amber started her own Instagram[6] page and put herself into a position where she gave others hope.

By chronicling her experiences, as do many people in similar situations, it had several knock-on effects. I have tried to get my head around, and will try to articulate, what they are. I think it is best summed up as it removed her from her own anxieties.

Amber had an outlet, a voice with which to allay other people's fears by addressing her own. As she experienced first-hand the good days and the not so good days, she was able to share what worked and what didn't. I guess it is similar to switching on a light bulb, rather than stumbling around in the dark, oblivious to the dangers.

From that connection with other people out there, either ahead or behind her on the journey, it gave her comfort.

I can understand that logic because, at the end of the day, it is about communicating.

---

6. instagram.com/unwelcome_breast_guest/

Over the North Atlantic, at night heading eastbound, I would sit there tuned into the common chat frequency all the pilots used as we watched the miles click down. Often, as a result of the jet stream, at some point in the journey there would be some clear-air turbulence.

The aircraft ahead would transmit their ride reports, as you followed in their trail, and you would listen out for these transmissions. If you heard "moderate turbulence" or "moderate chop" up ahead, you would brief the cabin crew, in case they were planning on going out with a meal service, and at the appropriate time turn on the seat belt sign.

So, what Amber was doing was "listening" ahead and passing down the line her experiences as she sailed into choppy waters.

A secondary effect, and one which immediately had an impact, was that it reduced significantly the number of well-intentioned calls to her asking, "How are you?"

Immediately, there was a "go-to" place via the World Wide Web and social media for friends and family to see how she was, good or bad, and have an update. It had started to exhaust her that she had to explain in minutia when there were days she didn't want to talk about cancer, didn't want to think about cancer and simply try to have a normal day.

It once again put her in control of the timeline, when she spoke and when she chose to have radio silence.

We are fortunate in as much as the people we call friends, both long term and those we have made in the West Midlands, are good people.

The last thing you want is negative people around you. One thing for sure is our friends are certainly not negative. It's absolutely true that the last thing you want to hear is doom and gloom; think positive, stay positive and once you have turned the corner there is hope.

Enablers is a term I have heard used as a noun in the United States, and it is only by checking Google and the Oxford English Dictionary for the word "enabler" do I find a definition that I have always associated with this string of vowels.

What I find is the two following definitions:

A person or thing that makes something possible.

A person who encourages or enables negative or self-destructive behaviour in another.

The word association I have, and one that I would harness as I moved forwards, is the former, and I would steer well clear of anybody remotely portraying the characteristics of the latter. The latter is always out there, however.

A person or thing that makes something possible is going to be vital in the days, weeks and months ahead. I would even argue that it is going to be plural and requires *people* to make something possible.

The light at the end of the tunnel doesn't have to be a train coming towards you. If you think it is, then step to the side, let it pass and keep walking towards the light.

Hope, after all, is eternal.

05 A Cunning Plan

Whilst it felt, on occasion, nothing was happening, it was.

A conveyor belt was being rolled out and Amber had stepped onto it.

Following an appointment with the doctor and a consultant surgeon, a date was tentatively set for her mastectomy and lymph node removal a few days before Christmas. As it happened, this was brought forwards to the 14th December, which meant that there was precious little time to do the Christmas shopping and get ready for what is a pretty invasive procedure.

Back under the care of the NHS, the surgery would take place locally at Warwick Hospital and, fortunately, our neighbours are nurses and immediately able to put Amber's mind at rest that she would be in good hands even though they would not be involved. A reassuring word goes a long way.

Appointments started to fill up the spaces on the calendar hanging up in the kitchen. There were pre-op assessments, blood tests, scans and even a check on bone marrow density that involved a trip over to University Hospital Coventry & Warwickshire to which I took her.

For all of the other appointments, Amber insisted on taking herself, something she was perfectly capable of doing at this stage.

Despite having breast cancer, there was no loss in weight, physical effects or lack of ability to function daily doing normal stuff. This helped, making lunches and doing daily chores, as mundane as it sounds, provided structure and, most importantly, a sense of normality.

Social media posts were starting to get a fair amount of attention, and the thing that jumped out was the amount of people dealing with the same challenges for cancers in the plural.

Colleagues who I had flown with were undergoing treatment for a variety of conditions including prostate cancer. My cousin was diagnosed with breast cancer at the same time and it felt like everyone was a victim of this "thing".

I booked myself in straight away for a PSA check (prostate-specific antigen test) and bloods to make sure I was not about to join the party. PSA tests help identify markers for things such as prostate cancer; though not perfect, it can be useful. Fortunately, they came back clear and, so long as something else didn't take me out of the equation, I would be available when I was needed over the next year or so.

The plan was fairly straightforward and was in effect in blocks: surgery... recovery, chemotherapy... recovery, radiotherapy... recovery, targeted therapy (one year) and hormone therapy (ten years).

I was learning fast, as we both were. The plan was to address the type of cancer and this cannot be over emphasised. Who constructs the plan? It is the oncologist, the consultant who is up to speed with the myriad of treatment options, and, believe me, there are a lot.

The type of cancer, it transpired, feeds off oestrogen, so remove it from the problem and you reduce the risk of reoccurrence. How you do that is either by medication, to shut down the ovaries, or physically remove the ovaries. Initially, the plan was to use medication. However, Amber made it clear she wanted to elect to have her ovaries removed at a later date.

This is hard for a woman in her youth to assimilate and something, fortunately, we did not have to face up to with four kids between us.

The mastectomy in itself provided options; reconstruct or not?

Apparently, they can do full reconstruction and even tattoo on a nipple!

Again, these are individual choices and can only be made by the patient and only their wishes should ever be taken into consideration.

Amber chose not to have reconstructive surgery, as she was concerned that having an implant, and in effect another "thing" stuffed back in place of the "thing" removed, would worry her for the rest of her life. In addition, she said she would look lopsided as she got older when the other boob sagged and the replacement was always on parade!

What's more, she was struggling with the health and condition of the remaining breast. If oestrogen fed the cancer cells in one, what was to say it hadn't done the same with the other and it was a ticking time bomb?

Well, in theory, the chemotherapy would take care of that and kill off any cancer cells, wherever they may be, including the healthy breast should they be lurking. Regular mammograms would also act as a safeguard.

She didn't buy into that completely and also found, post-surgery, that she felt "lopsided" and her fears had not gone away. It caused her unnecessary anxiety, worrying about the remaining breast, and therefore requested a second mastectomy that has currently been refused on the NHS as it is "elective" and not clinically required.

However, it transpires that some NHS Trusts support women's wishes to have a double mastectomy and some don't.

The gist of it is that this is something to be addressed further down the road and if it is necessary to go private, then it is an option, though not for all.

What I did not realise is that there are different pieces to the jigsaw puzzle, they are all choreographed, and the key to this smorgasbord is the oncologist.

One of the things that jumped out loud and clear in Kris Hallenga's book, *Glittering a Turd*, is that there are oncologists and then there are oncologists. The same as in any area of the medical profession, or in any profession for that matter, there are some that excel in their ability.

What Kris had to do, and something we all need to bear in mind, was get a second opinion, and even changing oncologists is an option. It's your life and you are making life choices.

As soon as a plan started to be sketched out, I could see Amber relax a little. Not to the point where it was time to kick back and relax, but it provided a framework, an order, a structure, and it started to put sense back into the chaos.

Was it set in stone? Of course not.

We knew that there might well be tweaks and changes to the plan, major or minor. There could well be new paths to be followed or just simply forks in the road where decisions would have to be made, left or right.

As Amber's partner and with my "checklist" style of professional upbringing, I found it reassuring that there was a plan. Sat there with an engine on fire that won't go out, flying away from the airport is never a good plan. Once turned around and going in the right direction, you can concentrate on the detail... survival.

06 Coping With Surgery

I didn't undergo any surgery... Amber certainly did and that presented challenges that I could never have foreseen at the time.

We both had apprehension, but it was Amber who had to deal with her anxieties leading up to the day of surgery.

She had a lot of anxiety the day before and, not surprisingly, didn't sleep great that night. Again, on the morning of her surgery, she had another wave of anxiety, and I always knew when she was stressed out because her hand, when held, was wet and clammy. The fear would literally ooze from every pore.

I dropped her at Warwick Hospital with a night-stop bag and off she marched. I was worried.

She later said that once she was in the ward and the nurses and staff engaged with her she relaxed, as they were all so friendly and cheerful. It was the waiting at home before the surgery that had been stressful, watching the calendar roll towards the day of the operation.

With it being a full general anaesthetic procedure and being knocked out, I knew it would be tough on her post-surgery and I was all geared up to microwave whatever she desired.

Amber, being Amber, had pre-cooked and prepared meals so that we could eat (not that we cannot fend for ourselves) and, once home, she could eat without fear of, "Oh my god, what are they doing?"

It was a long day.

They had said she may, or may not, be kept in overnight which surprised me. How can you have a mastectomy and lymph nodes removed from underneath an arm and be out the same day?

Apparently, you can.

The plan was to wait for her to contact me and I would return to the hospital to pick her up, possibly that evening.

I received a message.

All done and no need to pick me up as I am getting a lift home with Manjo [the nurse next door] *who has finished her shift and is waiting in reception for when I am discharged.*

With a feeling of relief, I waited and when I heard them pull up and I opened the door. I was greeted by a tornado, as Amber breezed in chatting away with tubes and a fluid drain bag, making straight for the cat's bowl to top up the biscuits.

Drugs!

She was clearly still on another planet and, despite the surgery, was walking along the ceiling.

After a short while, with the obligatory phone calls out of the way, she was tucked up in bed trying to work out how on earth she was going to cope for weeks with a drainage bag beside her without knocking it off, dropping it, crushing it or ripping out the two tubes connected to her. Something she was to do over the following weeks; not to be recommended.

But that evening, post-surgery, she went out like a light, tubes in place and the drainage bag intact.

The next day she was absolutely fine, she told me all about the day before and felt great.

The second day after surgery she certainly began to feel tired and slept for most of it.

The third day, exactly as the hospital had told her... *wham*.

The drugs had worked their way through her system and the bruising started to come out. Time now to concentrate on resting and, to be fair, she did.

A week after surgery, the dressings were removed and, being the brave woman she is, she had a look and was amazed at how neat the stitches were. It was healing beautifully. I tentatively asked and, to my surprise, she let me take a look. It was incredible to see just how quickly the body repairs itself.

Three days later, the last of the drains came out and that was a big deal, as it took away the baggage, literally. Celebration was a gin and tonic, on the basis that she had to replenish the lost fluids!

Three weeks after surgery and in the new year, she was doing really well. There was a reasonable amount of movement back in her left arm but absolutely no lifting or carrying of shopping bags was allowed.

There was, what is called, a little bit of "seroma" around the area of the incision, which apparently is normal, and, whilst uncomfortable, it is often seen until the body absorbs it.

Seroma is the technical term for fluid build-up. Even though there had been drains, one in three patients can have them post-surgery. Amber was one.

The big breakthrough, physically and psychologically, was the day in early January when Amber met with her surgeon, who gave her the news that he had got all of the cancer even though there had been a significant amount of lymph node involvement.

She was, as were all of us, ecstatic.

The "thing" was gone.

However, we knew that the cancer had been close to her chest cavity and, with all of the lymph node involvement, it was concluded that she needed to have, as she put it, the full treatment as a belt-and-braces approach.

It was time for a short break to recover physically before the next step on what seemed, at the time, to be a never-ending conveyor belt of treatment.

07 Wobbles are OK

Mental health has been rebranded to "well-being".

Which, to be fair, I can accept. For at long last, society, on the whole, is better at discussing mental health issues or pressures of life in a much more open and frank manner. Whatever it is called, it is important that it is discussed.

Men in particular, to be blunt, were, and in some cases still are, crap at talking about their well-being as it carries baggage. Masculinity, manliness and a stiff upper lip, moral fibre, backbone and "get a grip" spring to mind.

The reality is that we all have a tipping point and can have a wobble.

I often describe myself as being a pint glass that tries, on occasion, to squeeze in a quart and ends up overflowing. I believe, as I get older, that I am better now at recognising when I am about to overflow and back off.

Anxiety is often the trigger that we have to face on a daily basis.

The latest, with electric vehicles, is "range anxiety". Will I make it to the next charging point?

Anxiety can become debilitating to the point where it prevents us from doing something and can, in the extreme, prevent someone from even leaving the house.

Amber's anxieties and fears were right there from the outset, something to which she readily admitted. As a result of her open honesty, it then meant that the medical professionals had an opportunity to address these with mild medication and therapy.

But we all, to a greater or lesser extent, have fears and anxieties. Whether it is in our daily lives, or in this case navigating our way through the cancer journey, as a partner we too have stresses to deal with.

The overriding emotion and anxiety that occasionally engulfed me was the sheer enormity of it all. Not in terms of what I was doing, but what Amber was going through.

I was fortunate to have people around me, who were, very subtly, keeping an eye on me. They would look me in the eye and say, "Are you OK?"

The week before Christmas had been relentless. Amber had undergone extensive surgery in the middle of the month and had regular visits to the hospital to check on the drains and dressings.

For anyone who is not in the know, drains are literally required to drain off fluid that would otherwise build up following the trauma of surgery. So, as already mentioned, Amber had a plastic bag that continually filled, though less and less over the days and weeks following surgery.

This makes for extremely difficult sleeping and, as she pointed out, it is like having babies; you can't roll on them and you mustn't drop them!

But damage them she did, and as a result, field repairs were conducted late one evening to get through to the next morning where a hospital visit could put in place permanent repairs. The field repair involved lots of Sellotape and off we marched the next morning with her looking like she was a Christmas present wrapped up by a teenager.

The Tuesday before Christmas delivered another bombshell when my mother was diagnosed with bowel cancer.

I did not react as you would expect and just accepted it as fact. For weeks, I had suspected this was going to be her diagnosis and the only way I could prepare myself for it had been to accept it as fact before it was confirmed.

Getting your head around the fact that both your partner and mother have cancer is simply overwhelming, and I think I had just shut myself down to emotion in order to cope.

On Christmas Eve, Warwick District Council notified us, along with all of the businesses at the airport, that their planning officers had recommended the imminent approval of the planning application on January 11th 2022 which would ultimately result in the closure of Coventry Airport.

Again, I just took it as just another blow and did not flinch.

Christmas Day, we relaxed at home with the twins and my daughter. Without any alcohol at all in my system, by the afternoon I was wiped out.

I felt awful.

Lateral flow Covid tests were negative and my daughter, when I told her how I felt and the uncontrollable upset stomach I had, told me straight, "It's stress, Dad."

She was right; it had caught up with me. I felt pretty rough and after what was finally a solid night's sleep, I slowly started to bounce back.

Amber had gone down to her mother's with her sons in West Sussex on Boxing Day, as the boys can both drive, and my daughter stayed on for a couple of days with me before going home.

This period between Christmas and New Year is always an interesting time. It is a time when we tend to enter into a period of reflection, a period of respite from the world around us.

I found that with an empty house I had, not loneliness, but the space and capacity to think that I so sorely needed.

Leading up to Christmas had been intense, too intense, and I had neither the time nor the capacity to file things away into any semblance of order.

In the past, when I have gone on a hiking trip or a road trip, I have found it incredibly liberating to have the space to do just this, think; something we all need at different stages in our lives.

So, the conclusion I came to was that I had to be careful moving forwards and to make sure that taking "time out" was built into the cunning plan. It would be tough to rebuild any dreams, but this was one I would not allow to drift into a living nightmare. I continue to... love life.

Putting into practise what I preach is easier said than done, however. The trick was to carve out "me" time and the reality was it wasn't that difficult to do. There were days when Amber was too exhausted and was safely either tucked up in bed or catching up on the sofa with her favourite TV soaps.

I had always enjoyed the outdoors and walking or hiking in relatively remote areas had a huge impact in providing a relief valve from life's stresses.

When I flew professionally, I would often find myself in parts of the world that, whilst intense, were able to provide areas with an oasis of calmness, even in large urban areas such as Hong Kong, the last place in the world you would expect to find serenity.

Hong Kong harbour has, over the decades, slowly been eroded as more and more land reclamation allowed the city to expand and support its burgeoning population, but it hasn't lost any of its hustle and bustle as one of the busiest harbours in the world.

Hong Kong is a city of the senses, and the best way to experience the city and its diverse population is by walking. I must have destroyed a lot of shoes over the years walking its steamy streets and spectacular parks.

Aircrew are creatures of habit and, on the whole, have their own little routines in cities across the network, patterns that they follow and regular haunts that give them comfort.

In such a stressful environment, I needed a pressure relief valve, somewhere I could escape to, decompress and recharge for the flight back to London or onto Sydney depending on the trip's schedule.

For me, it was two places in Hong Kong, one of the most densely populated urban areas on the planet, Kowloon Park and Cheung Chau.

I would traverse the labyrinth of streets at the bottom of Kowloon, off Nathan Road, until I found myself at the park entrance where I would spend a morning free from traffic.

The first stop, with a coffee in my hand, would be the flamingo pond. Walking through what was often a fairly quiet and tranquil set of formal and tropical gardens, I could find myself in a different part of the globe and in a world of my own.

From the park, it is possible to walk across a skybridge and work your way onto the top of the Ocean Terminal, looking out across the harbour. More often than not, there would be large Chinese ferry boats connecting to the mainland and a cruise ship tied against the quay.

An observation deck leads out to the end of the terminal, with benches, where I could spend time at peace with the world.

Cheung Chau is an island connected by ferry from Hong Kong Island and is a fishing community with no cars other than the odd petrol-driven service cart on its narrow paths.

It was as close to a Greek fishing village as you could possibly get. It was a day out and always an adventure away from the heat and pollution of midsummer. As a result, I renamed it Cheung Chauopolis.

I am fortunate, because right on our doorstep, in the literal sense, here in Warwickshire is a network of walks, rivers and canal towpaths which lead me away from daily pressures.

It became my go-to safe haven, not Hong Kong's Kowloon Park or Cheung Chau but a way of coping when under pressure at home.

I was struggling with trying to file in my head and compartmentalise what Amber was going through.

At the same time, the world appeared to have literally gone mad.

For two weeks, we were all drowning in the rhetoric and politics of the COP26 environmental conferences at Glasgow in Scotland.

At the last second, India and China forced the wording from the agreement to *phasing down* as opposed to *phasing out* of coal. Nobody actually believed, however, that they had any intention of doing either.

Lots of backslapping, politicians in tears because of the enormity of having the world on their shoulders, as well as mankind's. Give us a break!

Meanwhile, Belarus invited refugees to pour into the country and guided them to the Polish border where they could enter the EU and have a better life. This being because the EU had imposed sanctions on the Belarus dictatorship as a result of its recent actions.

Thousands of desperate refugees massed on the Polish border as autumn had turned to winter. Politicians argued and, this time, it was the people who cried.

On Monday, the crew of the International Space Station had to take to their respective spacecraft as potential lifeboats, because the Russians had carried out a missile test and blown up one of its old spy satellites.

The destruction of the satellite caused thousands of pieces of space junk (i.e. shrapnel) to hurl into space and it was a little bit too close to the ISS for everyone's liking, including the Russian cosmonauts who were on board.

Living to the south of Birmingham and regular (or so it appeared) news of a shooting or stabbing by young people against other young people was also on the news.

I needed space to breathe and think. I could sense a wobble coming on, so I walked across the fields behind us to an old church in a tiny hamlet. From there, I dropped down the hill over open farmland to Saxon Mill on the edge of the river Avon.

A lot of the leaves had been stripped from the trees and swirled around as I descended. Ahead, I could see the old manor house and the cliffs which contained caves from medieval times with stories of murder and family betrayal. So clearly, the world was just as dangerous then.

I stopped and talked to a man filming the old manor house, as I assumed he was filming wildlife. It transpired he was taking daytime footage, as he had been involved in filming the night before for paranormal activity.

A "ghost hunter".

He proceeded to tell me how they had been in the caves the night before, which had been hewn out of the solid rock, and about a chair that had moved mysteriously of its own accord. All of this being recorded for a YouTube channel.

Continuing on my way, I took in the poor winter light and grey, sullen sky wishing for the warmth of the sun and bright hue of summer.

Back home, I found myself reflecting on the last few months and conclude that it had been complete and utter madness. The news feeds announced the rise in suicides and the deterioration of people's mental health, as a nation, over the last two years. No shit.

My son was in the Netherlands in a partial lockdown that looked more and more likely to go into a full lockdown, again. Austria tried to lockdown those that had not been vaccinated, quickly finding it was unenforceable and was about to go into a full lockdown.

The World Health Organization had warned of their serious concerns regarding Europe that winter. Just to add a further downer to the picture, speaking to the BBC, regional director Dr Hans Kluge warned that some 500,000 more deaths could be recorded by March unless urgent action was taken.

Oh, and to top it all off, the BBC pointed out that Belarus was a sideshow, because the Russian plan was actually to invade Ukraine sometime soon whilst we were all too busy worrying about saving the planet and a pandemic. To be later proven correct on February 24th 2022.

Tea helps.

With my hands wrapped around a mug of tea, Yorkshire Tea I hasten to add, the conclusion I came to was I could do bugger all about it. My priority, after supporting Amber, was fix the shed, tidy up the garden and make sure I didn't download a gambling app and blow all my life savings.

The good news being, I watched a TV programme on rewilding your garden and how important it is to make your garden as attractive as possible to the bees and butterflies, or anything, for that matter, that pollinates.

So just before I went for my walk, I ordered a "bug hotel" off the internet.

Proof, as if one were ever needed, that you don't have to glue yourself to a slip road off the M25 to Heathrow Airport to do your bit. You just have to pay the man.

It was no ordinary "bug hotel", I might add. It had enough compartments to not only provide refuge for anything that flew, crawled or hopped, but it had a metal roof!

No discarding it in two years because the roof has either rotten away from relentless rain or been eaten by one of the guests. No, a bona fide metal roof, just like the ones they have in Texas on ranch houses.

So, how was my mental health, my "well-being"?

Well, having been for a walk, and made a genuine effort to save the planet, I felt great.

It's OK to have a wobble.

08 One Step at a Time

By now, we were both getting into the swing of the journey and realised that you could only concentrate on the step in front of you.

Climbing a castle tower with a sign at the bottom saying "*Five hundred steps to the top*", whilst nice to know doesn't really help. In fact, it can be a hindrance and become daunting.

The result being that some people turn around and head for the gift shop.

The obvious difference with the cancer journey is that you don't really have a choice; the alternative isn't really an option. Therefore, by focusing on the step in front of you, if the steps increase or decrease in the future, you still reach the top.

The surgeon had competently done his part, a big step had been taken and the treatment ahead was, in effect, "mopping up" any rogue cancer cells that were gatecrashing the party.

Chemotherapy is tough on the body and, ironic as it may sound, you need to be fit to be able to take on the course of treatment.

The steps cannot be taken without the occasional trip, and Amber did have a bout of anxiety over the fact that there was significant lymph node involvement. The cancer care team have to be frank and honest throughout treatment, and they told her the truth that there was a possibility of reoccurrence later in life.

Once this was processed and filed, it was then possible to meet the anxiety head-on. The way Amber dealt with it was by simply resigning herself to the fact that "shit happens" in life and we cannot worry about things that haven't happened or may never happen at all. In other words, don't dwell on negative thoughts.

We were bouncing back and forwards to various appointments in order to have the growing checklist of items ticked off before further treatment could commence. This kept Amber busy.

There were scans for this and scans for that, checking organs, checking her heart was strong enough, bone density. It felt like a busy period, which it was.

Mixing in with the routine of pre-chemotherapy checks, we included as much normal stuff as we could by seeing family and friends.

Checking and trying out different bras and prosthetics is always going to keep any fashionista busy, and it soon became apparent that the fashion and retail industries as a whole catered for a lot of different post-surgery customers.

The Instagram posts were preparing Amber mentally with more and more correspondence with women who had gone through the next stage, often with the same type of cancer and diagnosis.

Suddenly the steps had handrails.

Looking back, through the power of twenty-twenty hindsight, I can see now how important the cancer care network is for anyone facing the challenges of treatment.

As a partner, it helped me tremendously. At the end of the day, I knew very little about the process and how to navigate through to a positive conclusion, but the people around Amber did.

At the same time, honesty is as always the only policy.

Accepting a rubbish day as a rubbish day often allows us to deal with it. Life isn't a wonderful, sun is shining and spring is in the air kind of experience. Our senses are heightened and enhanced to enjoy those sorts of days because of the rubbish days with horizontal rain and the central heating not working in January.

Amber made a social media post on the day of her forty-third birthday where she is full of joy, showered in cards and flowers. The big wins were the fact that her surgery had healed to the point where she could wear a hoodie again. The icing on the cake, as can be seen in the photo she posted on Instagram, was the fact that her lipstick matched the hoodie!

Cherish the good days.

The week after her birthday, she was back in hospital for an appointment with oncology to discuss her looming chemotherapy course and, most importantly, when it was going to start.

On that day, sat in the waiting room of oncology for the first time she posted:

Taking one minute, one hour at a time.

Remembering to breathe...

A date was set for the end of February to start chemotherapy and, needless to say, more pretreatment tests filled the calendar.

One trip to hospital was to have an "echocardiogram", not to be confused with an "electrocardiogram" or ECG.

The echocardiogram does indeed look at the heart and the nearby blood vessels, but it does it by means of an ultrasound scan. The appointment and scan doesn't take long at all and is, according to Amber (not having personally experienced it), painless.

The days quickly sped by, and we soon reached the day where I would drive Amber to Stratford-upon-Avon to start her chemotherapy treatment.

Time to take the next step.

09 The Chemical Sisters

"I absolutely don't want it, but needs must."

Amber's words and probably echoed across the planet by millions who arrive on day one for their first round of chemotherapy. So what exactly is it? How does it do what it does? There are lots and lots of questions.

The National Health Service in the UK makes readily available material covering a vast array of health issues. When it comes to the pages they provide, they are, as you will appreciate, regularly reviewed and updated.

At the time of writing, the NHS last reviewed the following on 25th May 2023 (source NHS UK). It therefore may be out of date and it is therefore prudent to check the latest publication using the following address:

https://www.nhs.uk/conditions/chemotherapy/

Chemotherapy is a cancer treatment where medicine is used to kill cancer cells.

There are many different types of chemotherapy medicine, but they all work in a similar way.

They stop cancer[7] cells reproducing, which prevents them from growing and spreading in the body.

When chemotherapy is used

Chemotherapy may be used if cancer has spread or there's a risk it will.

It can be used to:

- *try to cure the cancer completely (curative chemotherapy)*

- *make other treatments more effective – for example, it can be combined with radiotherapy[8]*

- *(chemoradiation) or used before surgery (neo-adjuvant chemotherapy)*

7. https://www.nhs.uk/conditions/cancer/
8. https://www.nhs.uk/conditions/radiotherapy/

- *reduce the risk of the cancer coming back after radiotherapy or surgery (adjuvant chemotherapy)*

- *relieve symptoms if a cure is not possible (palliative chemotherapy)*

The effectiveness of chemotherapy varies significantly. Ask your doctors about the chances of treatment being successful for you.

Types of chemotherapy

Chemotherapy can be given in several ways. Your doctors will recommend the best type for you.

The most common types are:

- *chemotherapy given into a vein (intravenous chemotherapy) – this is usually done in hospital and involves medicine being given through a tube in a vein in your hand, arm or chest*

- *chemotherapy tablets (oral chemotherapy) – this usually involves taking a course of medicine at home, with regular check-ups in hospital*

You may be treated with one type of chemotherapy medicine or a combination of different types.

You'll usually have several treatment sessions, which will typically be spread over the course of a few months.

Side effects of chemotherapy

As well as killing cancer cells, chemotherapy can damage some healthy cells in your body, such as blood cells, skin cells and cells in the stomach.

This can cause a range of unpleasant side effects, such as:

- *feeling tired most of the time*

- *feeling and being sick*

- *hair loss[9]*

- *an increased risk of getting infections*

- *a sore mouth*

---

9. https://www.nhs.uk/conditions/chemotherapy/cancer-and-hair-loss/

- *dry, sore or itchy skin*

- *diarrhoea[10] or constipation[11]*

Many of these side effects can be treated or prevented and most, if not all, will pass after treatment stops.

Please remember that everyone's treatment plan is different as is the type of cancer being treated.

The reason why Amber was being given a course of treatment (six months) was that she fell within two categories. It was being used to make other treatments more effective, surgery and radiotherapy, plus it was being used to prevent reoccurrence.

The plan being that radiotherapy, in her case would follow the chemotherapy.

There is a little one-liner tucked away in the above from the NHS that needs to be explained a bit more. *"The effectiveness of chemotherapy varies significantly. Ask your doctors about the chances of treatment being successful for you."*

---

10. https://www.nhs.uk/conditions/diarrhoea-and-vomiting/
11. https://www.nhs.uk/conditions/constipation/

The key to understanding what this means is the oncologist, the person who is up to speed with both your needs and options which are constantly changing within the world of oncology.

Amber would have the chemotherapy provided directly through what is called a "PICC line". This is a line that is inserted into a vein and feeds directly adjacent to the heart. The heart then pumps the chemotherapy around the body to reach every part of the body and tissue, within which a rogue cancer cell could be lurking.

It is a clever piece of kit, but because of the risks of infection having this attached for six months, there is something called "PICC care" scheduled throughout the treatment. In other words, servicing!

Ah... the bloody side effects.

This is, to be brutally honest, where I struggled.

The side effects are complicated and vary from patient to patient. The secondary consequence of side effects is that they often require pills or injections to address the main side effect, so a double whammy.

As a partner, and every partner and family member I have ever spoken to say the same, it is heartbreaking and emotionally draining. Nobody wants to see the person they care for deteriorating over time, day in, day out.

And that is exactly what happens.

The course of chemotherapy has gaps which allow the patient to recover sufficiently... to undergo the next session. Over time, the effects of chemotherapy and the side effects are cumulative.

Amber wanted me to drive her to all of her treatments and this I willingly did. I appreciate that some people choose to take themselves for treatment, but with hindsight, I am glad I took her.

The drive across to Stratford-upon-Avon is not an unpleasant one and, even though I would often be there for a very long time, it is a nice town to wander around.

The hospital itself was new, bright and airy. The unit, according to Amber, was a pleasant place to be in, with well thought-out treatment suites, big windows, music and staff that know how to lift the spirits.

Within the hospital was a Macmillan Cancer Support facility, staffed by volunteers, which was an excellent source of information.

I never set foot in the unit as another side effect, whilst undergoing treatment, is for patients to become immune compromised, so it wasn't only because of the fear of Covid being circulated. It is critical, therefore, to minimise risk of infection from everything and anything.

There is, however, a little cafe available on the ground floor and the hospital is very close to a canal towpath.

I spent many a day walking along the towpath, ending up at the canal basin at the bottom of the town. The river Avon meanders through the town with beautiful parks and the Royal Shakespeare Theatre on its banks.

In fact, as the year moved on and the number of tourists increased, so did my knowledge, to the point where more often than not, when asked for directions, I actually knew what I was talking about. If I didn't then bullshit baffles brains and I sent them off anyway with directions, hoping I wouldn't bump into them later!

The type of chemotherapy Amber was receiving initially is known as the "red devil", for a damn good reason. In fact, it is called EC (epirubicin and cyclophosphamide) and the epirubicin is red in colour, hence the nickname.

The chemotherapy attacks and destroys any fast-growing cells, not just those that are cancerous. This results in hair loss and has an impact on nails, skin and can possibly cause a sore mouth.

To address the white blood cells being compromised, a course of injections at the same time every day had to be administered at home.

These had to be injected into the fatty part of the stomach and Amber found it extremely difficult to self-administer, so I took on the role.

Our guardian angel Beq came around the first couple of evenings and demonstrated on Amber and then, under her supervision, I picked up the task. Once she was happy, and Amber was happy, I was on my own.

Amber became increasingly worried about my enthusiasm for the job, as she found the stinging sensation and side effects they produced uncomfortable. "Vicious little bastard" is how Amber described it. (The injection... not me!)

We always injected in the evening so that the viscous little bastard could do its thing at night.

We even had one of those bright yellow plastic boxes (a sharps bin) for used needles and big warning labels with words like *"Incinerate only"* plus symbols that were for biohazard that I had only ever seen in James Bond films at the villain's lair.

Amber insisted that the yellow box be kept in the garage so any visitors didn't think she was a junkie, something I told everyone she was anyway and that I was her supplier.

Every time I went down to the pharmacy, I would check I wasn't being followed and pop on my £1 Primarni, knock-off Ray Ban's. I only had one phone and felt a bit of a fraud not having a pocket full of burner phones.

As the treatment progressed, Amber's energy levels took a tumble and it took her longer and longer to bounce back, a bit like a tennis ball that doesn't bounce so high on the third, fourth and fifth cycle, eventually running out of momentum and just ending up sitting there motionless.

The thing that impressed me, however, was how Amber always came out of a session with a big smile and would tell me all about the interesting people she had met and how wonderful the staff were, plus there was the fact that they would have plenty of tea and biscuits, humour flying around and music to spice it up.

It sounded more like a social gathering than a treatment centre, and she said that was exactly the point; it was a place where people had hope and were surrounded by inspiration.

Positivity ruled.

After five and a half months, we drove to Stratford for the last chemotherapy session full of relief.

One thing we had been warned about, and one that we understood, was the post-treatment deflation that could hit Amber.

Having had, in effect, arms wrapped around her during the chemotherapy process, as soon as it finished she felt like a rug had been pulled away.

It was to take time for the body to recover and this was only in order to be strong enough to start radiotherapy. The comfort blanket was gone along with the tea and biscuits.

Keeping as engaged as much as we possibly could with friends and family had been important and was to be extremely indispensable as we lurched forwards to, not only more treatment but, the dreaded UK winter (as if summers aren't bad enough).

But thanks to Amber's tenacity, we kept positive.

10 Cool for Hats

If you want to get ahead, get a hat.

The side effect we all know about with chemotherapy is hair loss.

How people approach it and what they opt for are personal, and different people go for different options. The thing that I found amusing and reassuring was that this certainly wasn't going to keep a good woman down!

When we approached the beginning of Amber's chemotherapy, she knew what was coming and the NHS offered alternatives for her to consider.

First, and the most obvious, was a wig; something she looked at and quickly decided wasn't for her.

The other option was what is called "scalp cooling", sometimes referred to as "cold capping". This is where, prior to chemotherapy, a skullcap at extremely low temperatures is applied. It works by cooling the hair follicles to reduce blood flow and prevent or limit chemotherapy from affecting the fast-growing cells that regenerate hair.

It is only effective with certain chemotherapy drugs and would be discussed prior to treatment. It is apparently uncomfortable, for obvious reasons, and again, Amber decided against this.

Out came the scissors.

Amber had beautiful, long hair that she initially reduced in length as soon as the first hair started to fall out as part of the side effects of chemotherapy. She decided she was going to have fun with this enforced style makeover.

Next came a bob and then, very shortly after, it was an Annie Lennox-style pixie cut. The boys made derogatory comments about their mum's gender identity and it was quickly pointed out to them that they should be more inclusive!

Swiftly thereafter, it was the full-blown Sinéad O'Connor look.

Then, in a flurry of colour, out came the headscarves. Rosie the Riveter eat your heart out.

She now looked like a 1940s' factory, war effort poster girl and was determined to make a fashion statement all of her own.

The doorbell didn't stop as more and more scarves arrived; some generously donated by charities and some very kind retailers following her on Instagram.

Amber used to own a little shabby chic housewares and gift shop in Midhurst, West Sussex and always had an eye for fashion. There was no holding her back now, as every visit to the chemotherapy suite necessitated a new outfit and headscarf, brightening up not only her day but everyone's she came into contact with.

There are plenty of pictures on Instagram of her sporting the latest in headwear as the months rolled by.

For me, it was yet another example of positivity in the face of adversity; great to see and it was certainly uplifting for all of us on the outside looking in.

I have read so many times of people who are either going through treatment or are post-treatment adamant that cancer does not define who they are. I saw this first-hand, as the joy Amber got out of deciding something as simple as choosing a headscarf to match what she intended to wear made it normal.

In the streets and out and about, there was nothing self-conscious at all about it.

In fact, headscarves are a fashion accessory and there are plenty to view at festivals and events such as the Goodwood Revival; style never goes out of fashion.

Baseball caps were another option and occasionally would be the accessory of choice. Only classy baseball caps I might add; sassy all the way.

When we could, and it was always Amber's call, we went out and did something fun, even if it was a simple pleasure like sitting in one of the beautifully kept parks we have here in Leamington Spa.

I found it uplifting and always a joy to see a new headscarf getting its first outing.

If you've got it, flaunt it.

11 Onwards and Upwards

In between chemotherapy and radiotherapy come the requisite checks and tests once again, with regular visits to different units.

When Amber felt well enough, she would drive herself to either the Stratford Hospital or the Warwick Hospital.

As we moved closer to the day radiotherapy would start, more time was spent undergoing checks at University Hospital Coventry & Warwickshire, which, surprise, surprise, is located on the south side of Coventry.

I drove Amber to these appointments, as it was where radiotherapy was going to take place and, as a hospital, it is on a different scale altogether.

The first time we went there, I thought I was driving back into London Heathrow Airport and working my way through to Terminal 3. The only thing that was missing was the tunnel under the runway and the aircraft, of course.

It's a big hospital!

The buildings look like an airport terminal and are approached via two lanes, which route you through to a series of roundabouts, spearing off to more parking and buildings than you can shake a stick at.

The main hospital entrance leads you into a central foyer and opens up into a mini retail centre with shops and cafes. The only thing missing was passport control and duty-free.

The Arden Centre is tucked away past the main entrance and within walking distance from one of the car parks. It again is on a different scale to what Amber was used to and she found it a bit daunting at first, as the reception area was reminiscent to a departure lounge complete with gate agents directing patients to different venues.

As well as cancer treatment, they accommodate haematology (blood and bone marrow disorders) and have the ability to provide radiotherapy in a stand-alone unit.

The one thing we learnt very quickly during treatments was, if she felt up for it, regardless of what the medications were and what the impact was on Amber's general well-being and energy levels, we would use the treatment-free days to do something fun.

Friends fitted in with this on a day-to-day basis, so for Amber to meet up for a coffee with someone or for them to pop around would often be spontaneous and didn't have to be planned.

Since retiring from long-haul flying, I have kept my flying licences current and I have flown light aircraft on a regular basis, something I enjoyed doing, as well as instructing at Goodwood aerodrome part-time for a couple of years.

I was fortunate to have access to a light aircraft at Coventry Airport while it remained open. Every so often when Amber felt well enough, even during chemotherapy (usually the day before her next course when she had recovered sufficiently), we would go flying.

There are some great pictures of her on her Instagram page wearing a variety of headwear having fun.

One memorable day in particular, she felt well enough to go somewhere rather than just fly around locally. In her own words:

After a slow Sunday and Monday, I'm feeling good. I like to live big on the good days so we got up early this morning and flew to Shobdon Airfield for brunch!

When in the air, we can really see how lucky we are to live in such a green and beautiful country.

Unbeknown to us, a little hitchhiker flew into the plane while we were parked up. The poor little bee, all loaded up with pollen ready to take back to the nest, but it now finds itself in a different part of the country.

I remember that day clearly, it was a stunning day and one where we both felt on top of the world. We did the right thing and embraced it, putting it into the memory bank.

I think we both have the same values in as much as I am definitely a glass half-full sort of person. What I have consumed fulfils me and I don't worry about what is no longer available, I just look forward to enjoying what's in front of us; grateful.

Whilst wobbles are OK, banking fun days are important to keep it all in perspective; a bit like life really.

Onwards and upwards.

12 Walking in Treacle

No matter how hard we try, and no matter how many times we tell ourselves that wobbles are OK, sometimes it all catches up and some weeks are more challenging than others.

This is one of them.

Monday

The weather has changed.

After a long, hot summer, the air is damp and low-pressure systems sweep across the country, bringing with them a chain of storms that shatter the peace.

Looking at the weather radar app, it is easy to see the wall of red and purple, morphing across the screen, up from the Bristol Channel hugging the Cotswolds and racing across the Midlands.

Hopefully the surge protector will save my computer from frying should our little house on the prairie (OK, actually in a housing estate in Leamington Spa looking over a field) be unfortunate to be struck by a bolt of lightning.

The cat has decided to go into hibernation mode even though it is technically only just early autumn.

Schools and colleges have opened their doors, and I know the traffic will have ramped up exponentially and fully justifies my day at home working on an ongoing project, the return to revenue service of an airliner for a client.

Amber has chosen to drive herself to Stratford, to the cancer treatment centre, where she will be having a bone density scan. Today, she is adamant that she takes herself over and, whenever she is able to, maintain her independence. I get that.

There is an air of anticipation today, an air of hope that the country will settle down and stabilise into some semblance of normality. We desperately need "stability".

Today the new Prime Minister is to be announced.

Lunchtime has quickly come around, and the new Prime Minister is announced by the 1922

Committee (how very British and also fortunate that it is not the 1912 Committee, the year the *Titanic* sunk), the Right Honourable Liz Truss MP.

Phew, now we have a leader, I can get back to thinking about where on earth we can find a cockpit surveillance system for an aircraft that is out of production.

At 10 p.m., the heavens open and the biggest electrical storm of the summer hits the Midlands, providing relief, no doubt, to the water companies and stewards of reservoirs in the region. More sewage in the river Avon, of course, as the storm drain opens wide and disgorges.

Tuesday

The morning is spent reading through the list of parts that are slowly being procured, in preparation for the final push this week to get the airliner ready to fly again after its Covid slumber.

The new PM is on her way to Balmoral in Scotland to have an audience with the Queen as she takes over from her predecessor Boris Johnson. Boris is also going to Balmoral to resign and is no doubt hoping there will be at least one or two marmalade sandwiches going free, as he loves a good party.

We too are having afternoon tea and, with great reluctance, I have shed my summer shorts and T-shirt for something more becoming for a civilised event.

As part of our let's-get-on-with-life attitude and grabbing every opportunity we can to do fun things, we are going to "Whittle's" for afternoon tea.

Set in what was once a grammar school, and at one stage a convent, Whittle's is named after Sir Frank Whittle, pioneer of the jet engine. This is poignant for me, on a personal level, as I met Sir Frank when I was an apprentice aircraft engineer at British Caledonian airways... a very long time ago.

Sat in a grand dining room with a mountain of sandwiches, Amber is framed by two floor-to-ceiling, lead-panelled windows against which the rain lashes, interspersed with the odd flash of lightning.

She looks well and is getting stronger every day.

Wednesday

Amber takes herself this time to Warwick Hospital, which is only ten minutes away, for a thigh injection. There are no side effects with this one, and so it is straight around to her friends and into Leamington Spa for more afternoon tea.

Thursday

Today is a big day for both of us, as we are driving to University Hospital Coventry & Warwickshire where Amber is having her radiotherapy for the first time. It has been brought forwards, as we were expecting it to start next week.

As a result, we have managed to work out how we can manage the next forty-eight hours and achieve everything we need to. The plan sounds complicated and probably is, but I will drive to Portsmouth Harbour this afternoon where I will see my parents for the first time since February when my mother survived her bowel cancer operation. True to form, she is rumoured to be back to washing, ironing and feeding everyone who visits more than they actually need.

Beq is going to do the Friday hospital run back to Coventry.

I will stay overnight in Portsmouth and then my son, who is over from the Netherlands, and my daughter will visit us all on Friday afternoon in my parent's apartment.

Friday evening, I will drive back to the Midlands for the weekend, should there be any side effects from the radiotherapy, and then next Monday pick up the daily hospital run to Coventry.

That's the plan.

Having dropped Amber off, I find myself back in the hospital car park with an enormous box of chocolates in the back of the car for my mother and a large bar of chocolate as a medal for my cancer-kicking partner.

Amber appears and we swing back to Leamington Spa.

After a quick bite to eat, I leave for Portsmouth in the shadow of thunderclouds. Sure enough, it is not long before the heavens open and I am crawling along the A34 with the windscreen wipers beating as fast as they can.

The music on the radio is interrupted with news that members of the royal family are congregating at Balmoral where the Queen has been reportedly placed under care of her royal physician.

Rising and falling over the hills past Newbury, the wipers thud back and forwards with relentless rain reducing the visibility to what the police would probably call "poor".

I continue south onto the M3 and along the coast on the M27 to Portsmouth.

I soon find myself in my parent's apartment with the television on. We haven't even had a chance to exchange greetings when the news comes up, with a sombre tone, of the passing of Her Majesty Queen Elizabeth II.

God save the King

Friday

The news is dominated with the passing of the Queen.

I definitely need some air, as the apartment is, I find, stifling hot, something that seems to be a common theme in the homes of the elderly up and down the country. My father in particular struggles with arthritis and feels the cold.

After a brisk walk past the Isle of Wight ferry terminal, I circle around the fishing boats tied to the quay and cross onto Spice Island.

Once a den of iniquity, with pubs and brothels serving the fleet of the Royal Navy, it now offers fine cask ales, along with a variety of food and further beverages, with views across the harbour.

From there, I climb up the sea defences onto parts of Southsea Castle that provides uninterrupted vistas across the Solent towards the Isle of Wight.

Fort Blockhouse and Haslar, the former hospital, sit the other side of the harbour entrance. I brace against the granite walls as the wind blows through the entrance whipping up sea spray to add to the sense of drama, something only the sea can provide.

After a quick inspection of the new sea defences under construction, I head back to Gunwharf and the apartment where shortly my son and daughter will arrive for an afternoon of catch-up interspersed with a never-ending conveyor of tea and cake.

Driving back late in the evening, northbound, I listen to Planet Rock, loudly.

I find it reassuring to drown out the world and the madness, listening instead to sounds of the seventies from bands I grew up with. Emerson, Lake and Palmer are playing "Lucky Man"... how very apt.

Saturday

Back in Leamington Spa and conscious of Amber's first two treatments of radiotherapy, I suggest we go into town and have breakfast – not any breakfast, but eggs royale. You can't beat Scottish salmon with poached eggs and hollandaise sauce to start the day off right.

Back home and it is a day of chores. With the radio on in the background, regular announcements filter through of significant advances by Ukrainian forces on the city of Izyum.

Sunday

It is the Leamington Spa Food Festival and we spend the day soaking up the atmosphere, as well as more cholesterol than we probably should, in the immaculate gardens in the town we call home.

The war in Ukraine rumbles on.

The end of another week and a week where I have felt like I have been walking in treacle, struggling each day to put one foot in front of another.

We all have weeks like this; it is part of the journey.

13 Red October

With Amber slooowly getting her energy back after the chemotherapy sessions, we continued to do some fun things in between all of the appointments.

I kept a structure as much as possible to my week, with consultancy giving me the flexibility I needed to step in and out of the world of cancer. This was something that was, right from the outset, critically important for me in order to keep me sane.

Beq's husband and I have known each other for a very long time and we had flown long haul together, whilst at the same time he was a director of an aircraft maintenance company at Coventry Airport.

Steve is absolutely full of energy, always positive; "What could possibly go wrong?" being his catchphrase.

When Amber was diagnosed, he told me straight, "Amber is the priority for the next year." Whilst it was something I had already figured out, it helped to have someone you trust and, as a friend, validate your thoughts.

The truth is it is a lot longer than a year, as ongoing treatments are often in place to address different aspects.

The fact that her type of cancer is fed by hormones meant that it would require a monthly injection, to shut down the ovaries, of what is in fact a pellet that slowly dissipates over four weeks, along with a daily pill that reduces oestrogen production from around the body.

What it, in effect, is doing is medically inducing the menopause.

I will keep repeating myself here until I am blue in the face, everything I describe and mention is patient specific to Amber. It is based on her condition, her assessments and the guidance of her oncologist. It cannot be read across as a blueprint.

The "Zoladex" pellet injection, whilst daunting at first, is something she just gets on with now and is administered at the clinic, as it is way beyond my capabilities and I suspect is a controlled drug.

The picture of the needle next to a pencil on Amber's Instagram post made my eyes water, but she says it's actually fine.

By now, we were starting to get into the flow of life with hospital treatments and pills for this and injections for that. It started to become normalised in a strange sort of way, we just got on with it.

Silly little things that sound like a big deal were actually not; the wearing of a compression sleeve on her arm, for example, as a result of lymphoedema post-surgery[12].

The common thread, once the "startle factor" had been overcome and Amber had taken control of the clock (aka the calendar in the kitchen), is positivity.

Stay positive.

You will find a huge amount of material out there on positivity and the importance it plays in navigating to a positive outcome. Something I completely understood from my career as an airline captain.

As part of the role, people would turn to you in times of difficulty or stress. Leadership, no

---

12. https://www.nhs.uk/conditions/lymphoedema/

matter what you do in life, whether that's being responsible for a team in the office or managing a "crew" in a fast-food restaurant, requires you to stay calm.

"Oh my god, we are all going to die!" is not what you want to hear from the captain.

There is a time and a place for positivity, and a time and a place for a bit of me time, which is why, for example, ambulance crews and even the military have a network to support them in that way.

Our support network, and one we embraced, was our friends and family. Even though we had been in Leamington Spa for five minutes, support was there.

Amber never went to the "coffee mornings" that are available for cancer patients, and it is not to say that they cannot provide invaluable support for people. It was just something she didn't want or feel she needed.

The one thing I quickly learnt was to follow and not lead when it came to talking about it. I let her raise the subject, as and when she felt the need. It was not for me to bang on about it every five minutes. Besides, our dinner conversations when the boys were around were predominantly about the shortage of Lycoming engine cylinders and the safety aspects of entering aircraft fuel tanks with breathing apparatus and no matches in your pocket.

I drove Amber to Coventry hospital every day for her course of fifteen sessions of radiotherapy, with the one exception when Beq covered for me when I had been in Portsmouth.

Even though there were enough pamphlets and pieces of information floating about in the house, I must admit my attention to detail was pretty poor when it came to radiotherapy.

I know how radar works and I knew, as an aircraft engineer before I flew professionally, not to stand directly in front of an aircraft taxiing onto a gate in case they had inadvertently left the radar on and it fried my testicles. Not in the literal sense, I hasten to add, but long-term exposure, day in, day out to radar isn't good, hence the dentist always running out of the room, hiding behind a lead blanket, whenever they take an X-ray.

What I didn't grasp, however, is the fact that the dose applied, duration and where it is applied is completely different for each patient depending on what it is they are trying to achieve.

In Amber's case, it was a continuation of the belt-and-braces approach to making damn sure that any cancer cells that had escaped surgery, had escaped chemotherapy and were lurking in the chest wall were zapped.

Chest wall? Ah bingo, that explains it now, and when Amber spelt out the bloody obvious, I went a bit quiet – the heart.

All of these tests on her heart were for a reason, as the radiotherapy was also going to potentially impact organs behind the area being focused upon.

When it comes to accuracy, it transpires that she had marks (tattoo dots) applied to her skin for alignment so that each day the correct area was targeted. A bit like a surveyor, setting up a tripod on datum lines, is how she described it.

As you can imagine, the machines are complicated pieces of kit and it was not surprising that they would on occasions break down or require maintenance.

University Hospital Coventry & Warwickshire, as already mentioned, is big, I mean bloody big.

All of the hospitals we attended were different and had their own characteristics and vibe. Sutton

Coldfield was set in grounds with lots of trees and felt like it was in a leafy suburb. Being private, it felt like there should be Pilates classes going on and endless rounds of latte. It was a chilled and relaxed atmosphere.

Warwick Hospital is a hotchpotch of buildings all over the place, some new, some old, the mandatory Portakabins, and had the feel of an old army barracks. Straddling a road, there were car parks here, there and everywhere, ready to read your registration and send you a £60 fine because you got it wrong... your fault.

If there was one thing that I must admit pissed me off about the different hospitals it was the parking and the parking fees.

Nobody goes to hospital because they want to! It's not a leisure centre for goodness' sake.

Some appointments, in the treatment phase, were covered for cancer patients with a parking token, others were not. I suspect this too varies from NHS Trust to NHS Trust.

The issue I had with it was the fact that the vast majority of people simply could not afford the extra financial pressures and were being, I felt, penalised for having the audacity to require to go to a hospital and see a loved one every day.

The bean counters (no offence intended to accountants, by the way) will argue that it brings in extra revenue for the beleaguered NHS. I would argue that, as a National Health Service, fund it properly and have one CEO salary and not a CEO at every trust with their own management baggage.

Rant over.

Ah yes, where were we? Stratford Hospital. Very clean, modern, light, bright, uplifting and set around a courtyard with plenty of outside spaces including a covered entrance. It looked like it could just as easily be a corporate headquarters for an insurance company or a well-off local council.

Meanwhile, back at Coventry, we launched into what turned out to be, for Amber, a gruelling fifteen sessions of radiotherapy. There were weekends off, but Monday to Friday it was game on.

I found a way to the hospital through the back roads and pretty, little villages avoiding the main A46 that was, at the time, being ripped apart for improvements.

The unit has a drop off area and, initially, I would park up in one of the main car parks and we would walk across together, though, towards the end of the treatment, I used the drop off and would wait for a text to pick Amber up later in the day.

The sessions themselves were not long once Amber's name was called but, with backlogs and equipment breakdowns, we could easily be there for half a day.

Whilst the reception area was vast, the unit was primarily for patients, so I would wander across to the main hospital.

I was obligated to buy a bar of chocolate every time as a medal for Amber when we drove home, and I would treat myself to a coffee and often sit on one of the few benches outside watching the world go by.

The air ambulance would clatter in regularly onto the helipad above the car park that adjoins the accident and emergency department. Ambulances would come in and out and, on the ground floor, there was even a bus station, that's how big this hospital was.

It never ceases to amaze me how diverse a society we really are. If you ever need proof of that then a hospital is the place to see that up close, though the parking is a bit expensive if you ever fancy a visit.

You see all sorts and you have to chuckle, because some people clearly haven't got the message. There are signs everywhere saying *"No Smoking"*, *"Outside areas are no smoking, smoke-free zones"*. Nothing subtle about the signage but, as sure as eggs are eggs, I can guarantee that every time I was there, someone would be smoking away underneath one of the signs. Fair play, they might be there for cataracts to be sorted. Maybe not.

I even saw someone on crutches, with a bag of fluid on a trolley stand and a patch over one eye, in a dressing gown, stagger out, lean against a wall underneath a no smoking sign and proceed to slowly roll his own tobacco. Just goes to show, once a pirate, always a pirate.

It was a different world from Stratford, but I got to know the Coventry hospital intimately and, sure enough, it wasn't long before I started to be asked for directions. If any of you reading are one of these people, I apologise profusely if you ended up with an endoscopy when you only went in to see if you were colour-blind.

I was, as we both were, about to be caught out by radiotherapy.

I knew chemotherapy was going to be tough and, slowly after treatment, Amber started to get wisps of hair and tufts breaking out which lifted her spirits in the knowledge it might take time, but it would happen. Chemotherapy was starting to fade into the past. Radiotherapy, however, was the here and now.

The "targeted" dose of radiotherapy was intense, a bit like the microwave set on high as opposed to defrost.

Very soon, and as the treatment progressed, her chest area and around her upper arm became red raw. When I say red, I mean burnt, to the extent that it was worse than any sunburn you can imagine.

Here we go again.

Special creams and care to prevent infection were required, and it caused her a lot of discomfort. I confess here and now, I had a bit of a wobble, driving day in, day out and seeing her once again going through crap.

But not Amber, she just counted the days; number six, number seven... number eleven.

The treatment finished and in "Red October", she posted the following on Instagram, all very matter-of-fact and staying as always positive:

I completed 15 sessions of radiotherapy on the 5th October. Radiotherapy is strange, you don't see or feel anything. Just a machine moving around you and a bit of buzzing. That's it.

In and out in no more than 10 minutes.

I didn't appear to be burning until about session 13 when I started to go a bit red. By session 15 I was really burnt. It happened so fast. And it got a whole lot worse once radiotherapy finished. I ended up severely burnt and having creams and dressings prescribed. Today is the first day I've been able to wear a soft bra again!

So now I'm starting to feel like the worst of my treatment is behind me. It's a great feeling but scary at the same time. It feels like my safety net has been taken away. The calendar is no longer covered in hospital appointments like it has been for the past 11.5 months. No more regular banter with the nurses, radiographers or fellow cancer warriors.

In some ways I miss it. Isn't that a strange thing to say?!

Having said that, I'm just off to get my PHESGO injection this afternoon, number 8 out of 18. It stings. A lot. Wish me luck!

Bloody hell, Amber! I thought I was tough, but she was just powering through.

Behind the veneer, I knew I was wiped out with it all, and we decided to take off for the first time and booked a holiday.

It took a good month for the skin damage to sort of repair and a lot longer to fully clear. Mid November, we found ourselves on an aircraft first thing in the morning on our way to Malta, somewhere we had never been before. I had flown to most of the Mediterranean islands in the early days of my flying career, but never Malta.

We had splashed the cash and stayed in a very, very nice luxury hotel, kicking off our arrival with a bottle of Prosecco, for medicinal purposes of course.

Malta is hilly; the hotel was sat on top of a hill. Everywhere we went involved a hill. Bugger.

For someone who was in recovery a year on from having gone twelve rounds in a boxing ring, hills are not good. We soon learnt how to pace the day and enjoyed long lunches, sitting on promenades, using water taxis and limiting the Everest training.

It was, however, what we both needed; our first holiday since pre-Covid.

A lot had happened since then.

14 Don't Mention the "M"-Word

"Next mood swing in six minutes... be afraid, very afraid" is the sign hanging on one of the coat hooks as you come into our front door, given to Amber by our next-door neighbour when we all realised that medically induced menopause was going to be part of the treatment.

Monthly injections using what Amber described as a BFN (big f***ing needle) started before radiotherapy, so an overlap of side effects started to kick in with all of the treatments. Happy pills to compensate for the limited oestrogen production, the forced closing of business for the ovaries, meant I braced myself and bought a tin hat.

As it turned out, there was no need to, as Amber (and I can't vouch for everyone on the planet with two X chromosomes) didn't have mood swings or give me a hard time, that's for sure.

Menopause and perimenopause (the time around menopause when the ovaries begin to stop working) is a subject about which I do not profess to have a lot of knowledge. Suffice to say, the impact varies from patient to patient.

The big deal was what she was going through physically, and this manifested most dramatically with the hot flushes associated anyway with the menopause.

This was something, and continues to be something, that she has had to adapt to and address accordingly. Sometimes she is stood there glowing and flushed with sweat all over her face and arms.

At night, she struggled initially to regulate her body temperature and there is now an electric fan strategically placed at the end of the bed.

A delivery from Amazon resulted in what the boys and I thought were some latest boom box headphone gear but couldn't work out how to adjust them to get them over our ears. It turned out it was two mini, battery-operated fans that you slip around your neck and cool your face with.

Call ourselves engineers?

When I asked how long she had to have the BFN every month, she replied, "Oh, ten years or until such time as I have my ovaries removed."

We will just add it to the list then.

Amber learnt very quickly to listen to what her body was saying to her and adjusted the day accordingly, sometimes sleeping in, sometimes up and about early.

As the calendar rolled into another year, including exercise and relaxation became more and more of a part of her and, to be fair, both of our lives.

Swimming was the first big step, and we are fortunate to have access to a small pool that allowed Amber to build up slowly to more and more exercise, toning down what became additional weight.

Weight gain was to be expected with the amount of drugs and treatments that were applied. The first thing to do was to stabilise where she was and she did this by swimming. Walking was still limited due to joint aches and pains, whereas in a pool, with the weight being supported, muscles could be exercised.

As the pool is located in a small, private residential centre, there is also a gym with exercise classes and soon her weekly activities included Pilates and yoga, two very different activities concentrating on very different parts of the body.

The community Amber found herself now a part of was not a clinical one, it was social and, from that, she has made some new friends. Coffee after a class is part of the deal by the sound of it and, over the months, I have seen her spark come alive again and shine brighter each week.

One of the things that I was impressed with is her attitude to the enforced change.

As part of the treatment, there was a clinical psychologist available and the one area she didn't appear to struggle with was her self-esteem or identity as a woman.

With the hormone treatment and skinhead haircut during chemotherapy, whilst the boys joked about transitioning to being identified as "Trevor", Amber never took offence and laughed about it, as it was not a big deal as far as she was concerned. I can see, however, how some women would be offended and concerned about forced menopause.

It is not just in isolation, but a mastectomy can be an issue for some women, as can be going through the menopause at a relatively young or pre-middle age phase of their lives.

As the saying goes, one size doesn't fit all and I think partners and family have to be a bit sensitive and considerate during this period. It is too easy to get it wrong.

Yes, there were times when Amber said something or did something that I thought was a little bit out of character, but I certainly didn't package it up as part of the hormone treatments. I just put it down to, am I really surprised after the amount of drugs she has had going through her?

I am not qualified to talk or write about the impact on an individual; all I can share is my experience as an observer living with someone going through it. In Amber's case, it has been manageable.

If it does what is required and protects her in the future, gives her decades of life and happiness, then it has to be a good thing.

After all, that is what it is all about.

15 Kyle of Lochalsh

Leaning forwards, swaying with every pulse of the wind swirling over the ridge, the Isle of Skye stretches out before me surrounded by the frigid sea. I am breathless.

My stress release is walking. It always has been, and whatever it is that you do, hang onto it, whether it is cycling, swimming, jogging, golf or simply skimming pebbles on a lake.

Over the last few years, it has become my detox to what is going on around me. Walking was something that I had used when flying to clear my head, pounding Central Park in Manhattan or Kowloon Park in Hong Kong, it worked.

The sound of the communications mast behind me creaks and groans in harmony with the wind.

The Kyle of Lochalsh flows in its various hues around the jagged coast, from the sea loch over my right shoulder to Plockton sitting on the shore, as if it were a film set carefully crafted.

Far to my left, I can just make out the grey slash against the blue that is the Skye Bridge.

There is something unnatural about the view before me, for its natural beauty is overwhelming and I struggle to take it all in as it contradicts itself by its mere existence. I am overloaded and struggle to file each frame.

I start to break down what I am seeing into bite-size chunks, it is the only way I can consume all that is before me.

The backs of my calves are tight from the steep ascent through the forest. As I slip my rucksack down to the shale and scree at my feet, I can feel beads of sweat running down my back, this despite the cool breeze.

It is as if the stage has been set for me and all I have to do now is soak in the drama, the majesty and grace playing out all around me.

No sooner has a strap been whipped against my leg, the wind begins to die down and a silence envelopes the mountains, the sea and the sky. For I can begin to hear a dog barking in the distance, a train rumbles along the coastal track back towards Inverness, over two hours away. There's no more swaying of pine... just silence.

With the juices from an orange curling around my little finger, it runs quickly down to my wrist. I don't care.

It is a moment I have experienced before many times over many decades. I am back in the air and I am flying.

After what feels like an hour, but probably just minutes, the sound of scree being disturbed starts to reach up from the track behind me. Swinging around, I see first the top of a blue baseball cap and it is quickly followed by the shoulders and upper torso of a walker carrying a small blue rucksack.

Knowing he is not aware of my presence, I quickly call "Morning", as he strides around the base of the telecommunications mast splayed between us.

"Morning. Didn't expect anyone else to be up here in November!"

"Well," I reply, "with it being as clear as it is today, it had to be."

Immediately there falls between us a bond of respect for where we are, and we both just stand in silence taking in the view over and over again, absorbing the moment and etching forever the scene before us deep into our subconscious.

Pointing, he says "Skye Bridge" in a soft Highland brogue.

"No longer an island," I quip.

"Aye, you can say that again. Did you see the documentary the other night about the battle for Skye Bridge?"

Shaking my head, he continues, "If you get the chance it is well worth it, you should find it online on catch-up. It was a hell of a fight, but we managed, eventually, to get them to drop the toll charges... Got a bit nasty.

"I was warned off by the local sergeant who made it very clear to me that, as I held a liquor licence for my shop, if I was arrested on the bridge, it would mean the loss of the licence and I would be out of business."

"Blimey," I answer. "I will certainly check that out on catch-up."

Walking off the ridge and back through the forest, we talk about the area and the solitude and beauty out of season, the gridlocks of the summer and the dependence on the military for employment in the area. Deep-sea lochs have always been favoured by the senior service for hiding submarines from prying eyes.

Guessing we are both about the same age, we touch on time and its value, something neither of us, or anyone of us for that matter, grasps in their youth.

The connection with a stranger can sometimes break down all inhibitions and, with humility, he tells me candidly of his battle with cancer and another battle won.

Where the forestry tracks split east and west, we shake hands and bid each other well.

"Steve," I say.

"Paul," he answers, as we part and descend with our own journey ahead of us and another day, another moment in time carved into the granite of our lives, having met as strangers and departed as friends.

16 Good to Go

The day Amber was told she was clear of disease and good to go was an odd one, simply because she wasn't free. Or, I should say, she didn't feel free.

I understood exactly her sentiment, and there were all sorts of things whizzing around in her mind and mine, for that matter.

One of her posts summed up perfectly what she was trying to convey: "*Cancer doesn't end when treatment does.*" In fact, I would take that a step further and say cancer doesn't end when you are told you are clear of disease.

Whilst technically in remission, it's a bit like saying the car is back on the road after it has rolled a couple of times but now we have to get the dent's out and make sure it doesn't happen again.

It probably sounds a bit ungrateful but, in reality, there are some hugely significant things going on all at once and, in some ways, they are contradictory. I got it, I understood exactly how she felt, as I had lived and breathed it with her every step, as an observer.

There were lots of congratulatory messages and hugs from friends and family. Inside, though, I could see that there was a safety net removed whilst she continued to walk the wire, high up on her own.

Stepping out of hospital and walking back to the car the day treatment was over was a misnomer. Yes, "active" treatment was over but preventative treatment was continuing; the really important bit of making sure there was no recurrence, no relapse and no repeat performance.

After the consultant meeting where it was actually confirmed that she had the all-clear, Amber posted a simple one-liner:

Today we're celebrating being all clear.

No fireworks, no cake, maybe a glass of wine, but that was it.

I understood only too well, as my mother had undergone bowel cancer surgery, and because, I assume, due to her age had not had follow-up, belt-and-braces treatment as part of a preventative plan. In the back of my mind, and I knew in the back of my father's, the question remained: could it pop up somewhere else?

There is this expectation that a cancer story has ended and yet, in some ways, it is only just the beginning. There is a silence, a void, a feeling of departure and removal from the sausage machine that has protected you with all of its science and technology to defeat cancer.

Treatment, in reality, continues as, in Amber's case, the management of oestrogen, hormone therapy and medically induced menopause cannot stop. A future second mastectomy (Amber's wishes) and removal of her ovaries to remove the requirement for monthly injections all lay ahead.

In the meantime, in the words of another Iron Lady, many years ago "rejoice".

A mini break in a posh glamping pod in Wales helped, quickly followed by a trip to the Netherlands in the spring.

My son lives in Utrecht, and the weather was glorious, providing a much-needed bit of R & R.

"No bloody hills" was the criteria for this holiday, so we got that part right as well.

We had fortunately, or I should say, Amber had picked up on this part of the cancer journey and was mentally ready for it. Thanks to other cancer patients posting on social media, a lot had said that there was a weird sense of deflation.

It did not last though. Far from it, for as soon as the next stage was being engaged with, whatever "it" may have been, you are off again. You have just changed buses.

The twins turned twenty-one, so there were parties and places to go and people to see.

I was winding down my consultancy work and, as projects reached natural break points, I stepped aside.

We were both now good to go.

17 Chemo Curls

I had heard it mentioned but, to be honest, I never took on board what was really being talked about.

Oh, my word!

At first, when Amber's hair started to grow back, it was a bit hit and miss without really showing any definition or inclination to share with the world what it was about to do. When it got going though, away it went.

As I write these words, a year on from when chemotherapy finished, chemo curls are now in full bloom for the world to see. There are plenty of pictures on Instagram to see if you are so inclined.

A big milestone for Amber was when it was long enough for her to go to the hairdresser's and have it coloured and tidied up a bit. Whilst it sounds like not a big a deal, it is, believe me. It's all I heard about for a week.

Chemotherapy has a habit of altering the new hair and producing tight curls which, over time, will apparently straighten a bit, but by how much and when, we are yet to see.

For someone who, as we all know is a bit of a fashion diva, this opened up a whole new world: new clothes, headbands, make-up, you name it, it was delivered. And good for her.

She deserved it and it made her feel good, getting glammed up and engaged with the world again as an equal.

Every day, she would say that someone had made a comment about her hair. It certainly suits her, and the ultimate comment was when someone said she looked like Marilyn Monroe. Well there you go, result!

I have heard of incredibly courageous acts of kindness all over the world, where work colleagues or families "brave the shave" and join in unity with someone undergoing chemotherapy.

My hair is receding enough as it is, it didn't need a helping hand.

We were in Leamington Spa over a very short time frame, from February to the day of the diagnosis in October, and had hardly caught our breath when our lives changed overnight. Covid and being hit by the disease certainly did not help as we went through our first winter in a new part of the country.

A lot of people asked if we regretted having moved when events overtook us and we were removed, by distance, from familiar surroundings and friends and family.

The answer from both of us then and now is no.

We moved here for the right reasons; we are happy here and the distance is exactly that, miles. The reality is we can be in the south-east within two and a half hours, which for any of you reading this in the United States will laugh at. In Texas, driving two and a half hours to go shopping for the day is not unheard of. It's all relative.

It is sadly a bit of a postcode lottery as to whether you have a good NHS Trust in your part of the country or not. We are fortunate to have, based on our experience, what appears to be a good one. Not perfect, but that again is down to the people and departments you interact with.

I can at long last, slow down, draw breath and reflect on what has just happened. Today, Amber is out with her mother, who is visiting, and engaging in further retail therapy much to the pleasure of Leamington Spa's retail owners. I am going this afternoon to watch cricket at Edgbaston, near Birmingham, where there is both men's and women's professional matches scheduled.

I am not, or at least to date, a big cricket fan, but a friend from Leamington Spa has a couple of tickets and why not?

Last night, we had a barbeque with some neighbours around, and my son confirmed that he would be over for a long weekend in a couple of weeks. It is easy to run back and forwards from Amsterdam to Birmingham, so he will join us. The one request he has, however, is that we book the Millennium Balti in South Leamington Spa for the Saturday night!

The one thing I have learnt, and it is something we all learn in times of trouble, is what is important and what is not.

At the very beginning of this book, I wrote about the positive outcome of the treatment and the positive change Amber made by wanting to work in the medical profession by starting at the bottom.

Where someone starts is in fact immaterial, it is the fact that they are contributing and become a part of the solution that is really important.

Some people, post-cancer, help with charitable work, fundraise or concentrate on awareness campaigns. I don't think it is mandatory and it is up to everyone to manage their lives post-treatment based on how they see fit.

There are often high-profile, public figures who, when diagnosed, use their public standing in a positive way, something that a news presenter has recently done here in the West Midlands very publicly.

The BBC posted the following on their website:

> **_TV news presenter Nick Owen has revealed he has undergone surgery for prostate cancer._**
>
> _Owen, 75, well known for hosting shows including_ Good Morning Britain, _said he had been diagnosed with the "extensive and aggressive" cancer in April, on "one of the worst" days of his life._
>
> _"I was told that it was pretty serious and [I] had to do something about it soon," he said._

The BBC broadcaster is now urging other men to get tested.

Owen, best known as a pioneer of breakfast TV and his partnership with Anne Diamond, said he had had no symptoms and the diagnosis had "come out of the blue".

He revealed he had had a prostate-specific antigen (PSA) blood test which had shown slightly elevated results.

"My GP insisted that I go and see a specialist just to reassure me... he saved my life," he said.

The one thing I am not going to sit here and be, however, is be judgemental.

A lot of people choose to remain private and deal with cancer in their own way, behind closed doors, something we should all respect.

The chemo curls I see every morning remind me of how one person out of the millions who are diagnosed and treated successfully, dealt with it.

To me, it is a badge of honour... and, I might add, a very unique fashion statement!

18 Knowledge is Power

If there is anything that this journey of Amber's has taught me, it is the old adage that knowledge is power.

When I look back at the day when Amber broke down in tears in complete and utter shock and fear, convinced she had only twenty-four hours to live, to where we are today, it is absolutely incredible.

The key to successfully navigating, and most importantly, safely navigating her way through the minefield of diagnosis, treatment plans, oncology, chemotherapy, radiotherapy and hormone treatment was having the ability to overcome the fears.

This was achieved through knowledge.

Amber swears by the mantra of "question, question and question", anyone and everyone that she came into contact with.

From day one, in the room at Sutton Coldfield when she had just undergone mammograms, ultrasounds and invasive biopsies, she asked questions.

The nurse, on that day, looked at me and said to her, "Whatever you do, don't listen to him..."

"Oh, don't worry," replied Amber, "I don't anyway."

She was absolutely right.

The answers are out there and you have to seek them out from the professionals, not necessarily from friends and family.

What wound me up inside more than anything else was when people, innocently and meaning well, would ask, "What stage cancer is it?"

Ah!

People have this peculiar notion that being diagnosed with stage 4 cancer means it is not treatable. Not necessarily true.

What it means is that there are different treatment plans and different options, which the oncologist will work out. If you don't like the plan being proposed or have questions, ask. There is no reason why you can't ask for a second opinion, and you should if you have doubt.

As a captain of an airliner, I was not a sky god. I would constantly ask the other pilots for their input. It's absolutely critical in high-risk decision-making.

Don't be afraid to ask.

As a partner, this equally applies at different times and different stages. The caveat being, however, choose carefully who, when and how you ask.

There were occasions when Amber would come out of a consultation when she would talk all the way home, pouring out information, and would give me a blow-by-blow account of everything that was said. There were other occasions when she would sit there in silence.

It was never within my remit to then try and grill her about what was said if she was tight-lipped. It was usually because she was simply trying to process in her own mind what she had been told, and it takes time to assimilate what is sometimes complex terminology and dialogue from medical professionals.

If I needed to seek independent information, I would go onto the NHS website[13] as my first port of call.

I would, however, caution on using Google for everything, as there is unfortunately some whacky stuff out there. Dancing naked on the beach, whipping yourself with a rolled up copy of the medical journal *The Lancet* is not going to cure cancer.

In the UK, a good starting point is without doubt Macmillan[14]. The range of services and levels of support they provide as a charity is phenomenal.

Certain cancers tend to be pigeonholed into age or gender brackets... wrong!

Breast cancers, for example, cannot only impact women, it also affects men as well.

There is the mistaken belief that breast cancer is something older women contract and, as a result, checking for lumps and bumps, change in skin condition or discharge is not on everyone's radar.

Kris Hallenga, author of the aforementioned book *Glittering a Turd*, is co-founder of the charity

13.   https://www.nhs.uk/service-search/other-health-services/cancer-information-and-support
14.   https://www.macmillan.org.uk/

CoppaFeel[15]! Aimed at a younger audience, it has made significant inroads into awareness and the importance of self checking.

As already stated, cancer cuts a broad swath across genders and our bodies, bowel, breast, genital, skin and prostate to name but a few.

To this extent, it therefore means that whilst I have written about and described my experiences as a partner of someone who has had to deal directly with their diagnosis and treatment, it is possible to read across our experiences and give thought to where you are in the journey.

But without doubt, what Amber found was that the most readily available source of information was from the cancer care team. It was, obviously, by its very nature usually the most up to date.

Just simply asking, even about the machines and the equipment, helped her overcome her hospital anxiety and phobia. Incredible to think that two years ago the emotional wreck I held in my arms, trying to reassure, is now a clinical support worker in a hospital in an oncology department.

Science is working at an incredible pace and, whilst there will always be fear of the unknown,

---

15.   https://coppafeel.org/

empowered with knowledge you can smash it. It can be done and Amber has shown us all how, as have countless others.

19 Living Beyond Cancer

"Living with cancer", by definition, sounds like an anomaly.

In some ways, I guess it is. After all, who on earth would want to live with cancer?

The simple answer is we all would, if it kept us alive and provided a quality of life that we enjoyed, something that thousands upon thousands of people do every day. The one thing we have learned, however, over the last two years, when you reach that point, is to live beyond cancer.

Amber is adamant that it does not define her.

It is something that can have different connotations to different people depending on where they are during their journey. I apologise, by the way, for using the word "journey" on occasion, as you hear contestants often talk about their "Strictly" journey and this is definitely not a cha-cha-cha, darling!

The first exposure I had was when Amber was diagnosed, before a treatment plan was constructed and before any surgery or active treatment, whether it was chemotherapy, radiotherapy or drugs.

The biggest stress factor for Amber, and something she shared, was the knowledge that this "thing" was in her body and she wanted it out, gone, cut out as soon as possible, in the bin (read incinerator) and out of the equation. Even though, as was pointed out by the cancer care team, the lump/tumour had been growing for a long time, waiting a few weeks before surgery, in their opinion, was not going to make any difference.

Well, actually, even though I am not a healthcare professional, it does.

Amber and I knew that the cancer cells had spread to her lymph nodes in her left arm and, until they were removed, it could not be determined if they were all infected. If they were all infected, it could have progressed to other parts of her body.

So, whilst it is great to have a plan, it doesn't necessarily remove all of the fears and anxiety from the situation. We were afraid of the clock.

How did we cope?

To be honest, at that stage we were along for the ride and were in no fit shape to have a new norm in our new world of hospitals and treatment. The truth is we just bumbled along until the day of surgery.

Following surgery, the next thing we had to live with was the time it takes to get the results from the material removed. Was the mastectomy a clean removal with no cancer cells on the chest wall margins? Were all of the lymph nodes involved?

The results when they came, as already mentioned, gave Amber confidence that the "bloody thing" was physically out of her body and not able to do its evil work.

We knew a lot about what lay ahead, as there was a lot of guidance and information provided by everyone that Amber came into contact with; not too much information but enough to take on board where we were.

It is fair to say, at this point, that we are all different, and some people choose not to know too much, show up for appointments and go home. We really are all different and how you or the next person deal with it is up to the individual. You make your own path and do what is right for you.

We, however, are both information bandits. My technical background probably means I can take on board the vast majority of what is being thrown around. Amber's appetite for information was her coping mechanism; the more she found out the more she felt like she was in control and not sat in the back seat.

At home, the boys had, by now, started to get their heads around what was going on, as had parents, extended family and friends.

The communication outlets used by Amber (Instagram and Facebook) proved to be a godsend, because it managed everyone's appetite for information and reduced significantly the number of calls. It also allowed her to do at least something while resting up post-surgery and waiting for the next consultation.

I used the time at home, when Amber was recovering, to step out of the world we found ourselves in and concentrate on managing projects for clients remotely.

The beauty of working from home is the fact that, if you have the discipline to turn it on and turn it off, you can live in parallel universes, something that certainly helped me, without any shadow of a doubt, shut away from the changes that had been forced upon us.

One thing we didn't do, and is something that I have to stress, was wallow in self-pity. Amber certainly did not, and I just dealt with it in a mechanical, building block fashion, moving from one phase to the next, adapting as required.

During this period, as previously mentioned, my cousin was diagnosed with breast cancer and my mother was about to go into surgery for bowel cancer. We were not the only ones dealing with challenges.

The Instagram page Amber had set up had opened up a world we didn't know existed, and our little world in the big scheme of things was not that big a deal compared to what other people, their families and loved ones had to face up to.

During the chemotherapy phase of the treatment, the biggest change in our lives was Amber's fatigue. The thing to remember here is the reality of the timeline between chemotherapy sessions. It is for one purpose only, and that is to allow the chemotherapy to spread with consistency and for the patient to recover sufficiently for the next session.

So what we started to see was a cycle, where a few days after the chemotherapy session fatigue would set in and there would be a low point where Amber was wiped out and then would slowly get her strength back and then, the day before the next session, she would be able to get out a little bit. It was usually the day before a session we would try to do something fun.

I must admit, towards the end of the five and a half months of chemotherapy, I started to suffer from battle fatigue. It wasn't the driving back and forwards to the hospital, but it was having seen a vivacious woman physically beaten down over time with the constant battering her body had taken, in order to make her better.

It was probably, for me, one of my low points. I felt useless, helpless and, I guess, a bit of survivor's guilt because I wasn't going through this but was watching.

Seeing someone you care for, day in, day out, going through the chemotherapy process is without doubt hard for a partner.

The other overriding memory I have of chemotherapy is the smell.

I could smell it oozing from her skin at night and it is a peculiar metallic, like an iron ore forge, blacksmith's smell, or at least that's what it smelt like to me. It took a while to dissipate after treatment, but I am relieved to say that when I woke up, there wasn't a medieval suit of armour morphed over her body!

I have already touched on the injection side of it, but injecting into Amber's stomach is something I was able to do, but it is something I am glad was finally behind us once the course was completed.

Thank goodness for video calls on our all-singing, all-dancing phones these days.

Amber was able to communicate with family and friends when she wanted to and would go to great pains to put on a bright headscarf and doll herself up a little bit, something that I am sure was reassuring for everyone who harboured their own concerns, putting on a brave face.

By the same token, I was very mindful and careful to be positive whenever someone asked, "How's Amber?" Amber is, was and always will be, a positive person and brings positive energy into a room. Negativity just isn't part of her vocabulary, so the last thing I wanted to do was cast a shadow on that.

We soon fell into a routine with household chores, and even now, I do the jobs that require any serious mobility, vacuuming, ironing and carrying bags. This is because of a combination of drugs that have side effects restricting mobility and the lymphoedema as a result of the surgery.

Having treats is important, and Amber found that because of the impact on her taste buds she suddenly developed an insatiable appetite for Chinese food. As a result, we ate a lot of Chinese food and could probably write a guide on Leamington Spa's finest Chinese cuisine.

Chocolate became a staple as well, and I was never allowed to go out shopping without bringing back a bar, the larger the better.

Radiotherapy was a surprise, based on the extent to which it burnt and immobilised Amber, causing discomfort.

We thought that this part of the treatment would be easy compared to chemotherapy, but we underestimated the impact it would have on day-to-day living. In short, it does, and it was things like wearing a seat belt, sat in the left-hand seat as a passenger (UK), she had to get her thumb under the belt to give sufficient clearance away from the burnt skin.

In the right-hand side, driving? No chance. So there was no driving for Amber at all during that period and, to be honest, with chemotherapy taking an incredibly long time to get out of her system, it was probably not a bad thing.

We certainly clocked up the miles and one thing I would say is if, as a patient, you are fortunate to have someone to drive you to hospital appointments, take advantage of it.

I appreciate there are many, many people who drive themselves to hospital simply because they have to, but if you can afford a taxi or a bus is available, use them. It just means that there is one less pressure, one less piece of stress added to the pile.

There is definitely an uptick in energy and spirit once the radiotherapy and its effects are complete. I could see Amber, over the days and weeks, bounce back. Whilst it seemed to me to be slow, other people could see her spark coming back.

Her Instagram page[16] shows that clearly in the pictures over time.

Friends and family make up a tremendous part of how someone lives with cancer.

16. https://www.instagram.com/unwelcome_breast_guest/

Right from the word go, Amber was showered with love and affection, quite rightly so, which in itself is a medicine.

This is probably well worth expanding upon.

I have endeavoured to write, throughout, a partner's perspective and that of the family. The person at the centre is the patient, in this case, a cancer patient. What has dawned on me, however, is that the emotions and challenges I have faced can be equally applied to someone supporting someone with other life-changing events.

There are events such as bereavement, life-changing injuries or disabilities that, when faced by a family, have to be overcome. Yes, it is important to provide love and support to the person at the centre, but it is equally important to include each other. In other words, include those who are on the outer ring.

We knew before all this kicked off that our move to the West Midlands was the right one for us, because of the people.

It came to the fore when, after having lived here for only six months, overnight, neighbours became and remain good friends. The generosity and compassion they showed us has been humbling.

Included in this is everyone I had a professional relationship with at Coventry Airport. In particular, the good people at AeroTech Aircraft Maintenance who wrapped their arms around one of the boys, whilst his mum was going through treatment.

It took the pressure off me and, for that matter, Amber as well, because when he went to work every morning, we knew that he was being kept busy and his mind was occupied surrounded by his work colleagues.

His twin brother, because he works at Farnborough Airport, lives with his dad in West Sussex, would more often than not spend the weekend with us and, again, it was something that would lift Amber's spirits, having her boys around, even though they are adults and can drink me under the table!

The doorbell would ring and, more times than not, when opened, a neighbour would be stood there with flowers, cakes or Indian home-made pakoras.

Even when the "all-clear" or, to be technically correct, you are told that at that particular moment in time you have no evidence of disease (NED) preventative treatment continues, whether it be injections, pills or hospital visits for scans, there is still a structure and regime.

So in that sense, in my mind, we are still living with cancer.

Amber has ahead of her further surgery – ovary removal to prevent the body from generating oestrogen and an elective procedure for a second mastectomy.

The second mastectomy will be her choice and one everyone has to make as an individual. In her mind, she argues that whilst knowing the breast that developed cancer cannot spread it any more, she fears that later in life the remaining breast could. So, therefore, she doesn't want that angst.

In addition, she feels lopsided and unbalanced and would rather just be flat.

What do I think?

Well again, as I have said over and over again, as a partner, I see my role as primarily being supportive and it is for people to make personal decisions based on their wishes, not somebody else's.

Do I think it makes a woman any less of a woman or less attractive? Absolutely not.

Does Amber sometimes make me roll my eyes and go... OK! Of course.

Recently, we have been doing more and more fun things, despite the all-time poor British summer. We were well and truly beyond cancer in our minds and in our conversations. Downtime has been our time.

One of our neighbours invited Amber to go with her to Belfast for the weekend, as she had a friend who had an engagement party planned.

So on a Saturday morning at double "O" early, I drove them to Birmingham Airport, gave her a kiss and said, "Have fun, see you tomorrow night."

Game on for some me time and the opportunity to try and give the cat some "one-to-one" counselling.

Sunday evening, as I settled into a bit of television, I checked the progress of the flight back from Belfast and I saw it was delayed an hour so sat back and relaxed.

Just as the obligatory *Countryfile* came up on the telly, I double-checked the calendar, as I hadn't heard anything from Amber and just put it down to a hangover and shopping.

Yep... Saturday and Sunday... Northern Ireland.

Deciding brownie points in the bag were always worth having, I headed up to the airport. Based on the time of arrival, and allowing thirty minutes for bag collection, I should be able to swing into the pickup area, pay the obligatory parking fee, pick them up and head home.

Ten minutes from the airport, I still hadn't received a *"Landed"* text, so I pulled into a lay-by and sent a text saying, *"Hi love, I'm 10 minutes away in a lay-by."*

A sixth sense started to kick in, so I called... No answer... Must be still on the aircraft or going through the cattle crush and can't hear the phone.

Forty-five minutes later in the lay-by with people slowing down as they went past convinced I was in an unmarked police car... nothing.

Second text... *"Hi love... Do you have your bags?"* Still nothing... Second call, no answer.

Mmm. Processing everything on the hoof, I decided to drive into the airport, pay the man and see if they were there with two flat batteries in two mobile phones... Possible?

Just as I started the engine to resume my journey, my phone rings... Amber.

"Did you try to ring me?"

"Yep, I am ten minutes away. Have you got the bags?"

"We've just come out of the cinema and are walking back to the hotel."

Needless to say, they were still in Belfast and were coming home in twenty-four hours' time... not that night.

For a nanosecond, as I frightened other road users going all the way around a roundabout and back the way I came, I was not a happy bunny.

Then I laughed out loud, as it was the Amber I knew and loved because it was "obviously" my entire fault. Did it matter? Of course not. They were safe, she was having a girly weekend and tomorrow there were no planned hospital visits.

I blame the drugs.

Footnote: Amber and Manjo are adamant I just didn't listen!

20 Swiss Cheese

I am staring at my phone, dreading what is about to happen, when I eventually open up the message from the medical centre.

I am sat in my parent's apartment having driven down from Leamington Spa. To my side, through the double glazing, I can hear the sound of dozens of car alarms, as the Isle of Wight ferry leans into a sharp turn to exit Portsmouth Harbour.

I just stare at the leather cover on the phone and, with that, it pings again to remind me that I need to open it, read it and accept my fate.

How the hell did this happen? How did I get into this predicament?

It is late August and it is the last bank holiday we have until Christmas. So it is a long weekend, with the city heaving as people pour in to attend the

"Victorious Festival" along the sea front. I neither feel victorious nor festive.

My journey started back in the spring when I flew to Halfpenny Green (pronounced Ha'penny Green and, yes, it is another real, quintessentially British name).

I had not paid a visit to the restroom before the flight and, even though a short flight, by the time I arrived I was bursting for the toilet.

I made it without embarrassment and there, to my horror as I strained, was a small amount of blood in my urine, staring back at me, saying... "OK smart-arse, what are you going to do about that then?"

Don't panic was my immediate thought as I had heard of this before, and I had without doubt been straining to control my bladder and it might just be nothing.

On the other hand, it might be something...

Over the following days, there was absolutely nothing, no blood, no pain, no strain, it had never happened before and had disappeared, so it was probably nothing to worry about.

But I did worry.

I knew that blood in urine is a potential symptom of all sorts of nasties, prostate, liver and the list goes on.

I peed probably more often than, say, a twenty-year-old that is blessed in youth with the bladder of a camel. The only way I was going to sort this out and put my mind at rest was to arrange for a health check.

As it so happened, I was due one anyway as part of the NHS over sixties, "let's check you out" health checks.

I called the medical centre and explained that I wanted to book a blood test and a follow-up appointment with my doctor. I explained about the one-off blood in the urine and I asked if I could have a PSA check for possible prostate cancer.

"Absolutely," was the reply, "and we will book you in for a double doctor's appointment." Whoopee, twenty minutes instead of ten.

I felt good; I was on top of it and would quickly know if I really had something to worry about or not.

Having spent the last couple of years seeing what Amber had gone through, having read all of the literature and been bombarded by public service messages on the TV and radio... I understood. Get it checked early. The earlier the diagnosis, the earlier the treatment, the better the survival rate.

A week after the blood was taken, I walked right across town to the medical centre and topped up my step count as part of my "let's drive less and walk more" mindset. Thanks of course to Greta.

My name flashed up on the screen, and I knocked on the door before entering. As I entered, I immediately spotted a second person sat to the right of the doctor with a file, papers and a smile.

Shit, there's two of them.

Shit, I knew all about this, I remembered being dragged out of the car in a car park, at Sutton Coldfield, to listen to Amber being told, "We think it possibly... but wait for the biopsy... at least a year if treatment is required."

My heart sank.

"Good morning, this is Nurse Armageddon and she is here as part of her training to observe me today."

(OK, her name wasn't Armageddon, but I had already made my mind up.)

Looking at the screen the doctor said, "Have you got your blood pressure ticket?"

"Sorry, blood pressure ticket?" I responded.

"Ah, OK. Go back to reception and at the entrance is a room with a blood pressure machine. Follow the instructions and bring it back to me, please."

Like a lamb to slaughter, I shoved my right arm all the way into the machine, pressed start and waited for it to do its boa constrictor deed and spit out a ticket.

Back in the doctor's surgery, I handed over the ticket and immediately saw her eyebrows go up. I wasn't sure if I was about to be pushed off the chair and have paddles thrust onto my chest, or I had simply pressed the wrong button and had a printout of that month's electricity usage for the entire medical centre...

"Statins," she said.

"Statins?" bleated I.

"I don't like your blood pressure reading, your cholesterol is higher than it should be and, according to this algorithm, you have a chance of a heart attack and statins will reduce your risk." The doctor paused.

My brain was processing all of this in overdrive. So, no mention of PSA, prostate markers or cancer, we were talking about general health and, like everyone over sixty, I was being pushed toward statins.

I now composed myself, as the fear I had walking in, with prostate cancer, had disappeared.

I started to engage and realised I had just walked several miles, shoved my arm into a machine with only one blood pressure reading, coupled with the fact I was probably eating more crap than I should; I could actually do something about this.

I fought my corner and it was agreed that I would spend the next three months concentrating on what I ate, volume and quality, swimming more, walking more and cutting out caffeine. As a British male, my entire molecular make-up of H_2O was actually tea.

I left that morning elated. Nurse Armageddon was in fact a newbie nurse, I probably needed a kick up the backside in terms of what I ate, something I could tackle, but most importantly, nothing was mentioned about the PSA markers being high. Result.

I kept to my side of the deal. I did not want statins and if I could apply a bit of discipline then I could avoid them moving forwards.

I immediately went decaf with tea and coffee, something that impacted me in a positive way with sleeping.

I ate less junk food and snacks and more fruit, a lot more fruit. The noticeable change there was the obvious one and I felt better as each week went by.

Alcohol, while never being high in terms of consumption, was swapped out with alcohol-free beers, which incidentally have come a long way and no longer taste like dishwater.

The deal was that in three months I would have another blood test. A week later, I would have a "single", ten-minute doctor's appointment and we would see how I had got on.

I was just as much intrigued as the doctor to see if I had whipped this into shape and, following a blood sample the week before last, on Monday of this week, I found myself sat in front of the doctor, on her own, smiling. We were both smiling.

Blood pressure down, cholesterol down and both were in very normal, safe areas on her screen. Tick.

I felt good and I said, "That's a relief, I must admit I was pretty stressed when I came here in May, as I was more worried about the PSA result having passed that little bit of blood in my urine."

She looked at me and said the one thing you don't want to hear, "What blood in your urine?"

My heart sank and I said, "The one occasion I had a little bit of blood which I explained in detail when I made the appointment to have the blood test and specifically requested the PSA check for."

Her fingers were flashing across the keyboard and simultaneously she said, "There is nothing in your notes!"

Without drawing breath, she continued to say, "The PSA check back in May was fine."

"Oh, that's good," I croaked.

Before I could make a bolt for the door, she said "I want you to do a urine test" and started to pull labels and a bottle along with a bag out of a cupboard.

"We are going to test for red blood cells and see if there is any blood in the urine that is no longer visible, as there could be something going on, even though you no longer see it."

I sat for half an hour in the waiting room drinking water so I could fill a small plastic bottle, in the toilet I might add. There'd been too much stress for one day, being arrested and upsetting the good people of Leamington Spa was not a good idea.

With the specimen in a clear plastic bag for the world to see, I handed it over the counter without having to queue. Everyone parted to let me through for some reason.

I stepped outside, having been told, "If you don't hear from us it is OK."

Bloody marvellous.

I was angry. Angry at the fact that a cock-up had occurred when I called back in May and the critically important piece of information, the blood in the urine bit, had not been put on the appointment details. As a result, it had become a "health and welfare check" for someone in their sixties.

I was angrier, however, with myself. The holes had all lined up in the Swiss cheese and now I was at risk of having lost three months if there was actually a problem.

So having just gone through Amber's journey, I had two problems, both of which were, to be honest, of my own doing. I had lost control of the clock for three months and put myself in an "at risk" position until the results came back.

The "Swiss cheese" analogy is used in high-risk environments to describe what happens when you are trying to prevent something getting through and then the holes in the Swiss cheese all line up one day and "it" gets through. In aviation it means crashing. The first thing you learn as a pilot is don't crash.

I don't blame the medical centre, I blame myself.

It was a Monday afternoon and Amber's mother was visiting. The plan being that I would take her at the end of the week, on Friday morning, south and continue on to Portsmouth and check on my parents.

My mother is going through more tests and checks, as they have concerns over a recent MRI scan. I try to visit monthly and, as it so happens, I planned on going down this week anyway.

Tuesday, this week, came and went with no news.

Wednesday afternoon my phone rang in the afternoon and, sure enough, it was the medical centre.

"Can you come down and collect a red-topped specimen bottle that the doctor wants you to fill tomorrow morning, get back to us before midday and the laboratory will analyse it in the afternoon."

Now I was worried; a second sample to be analysed the same day, with a big, red, urgent lid and paperwork, most of which were barcodes.

Yesterday morning, on Thursday, at one minute past eight in the morning, I handed over the specimen to the receptionist knowing that Friday would be "D-Day". Assuming it was analysed as planned in the afternoon, the results would be back Friday. Again, I was told that they would only call me if it was necessary, their logic being that with hundreds of results each day, they couldn't call everyone but, if next week I was concerned, I could call them.

Amber calmed me down and said, "Chances are it's nothing and they are covering their backsides with all of these tests, as it's what should have happened three months ago."

This was weird. Now my partner, who is a cancer survivor, was reassuring me, as I sat in limbo waiting for the results. I appreciated what she was saying and suddenly felt the anxieties she felt, what feels now, a lifetime ago.

Today, I drove to Midhurst in West Sussex, dropping Amber's mother off and, after lunch with some good friends, continued on to Portsmouth.

Now, I am staring at the phone and, with my parents sat at the table, I open the message:

Dear Mr. Ford,

Just to let you know that your recent urine test has been reported as normal with nothing for you to be concerned about.

Best wishes.

Time to breathe and it is time to get on with life.

"I really believe this and the source of art is love. I love life." – David Hockney

21 The Important Part

This is probably the most important part of the book!

Not because I want to list the hundreds, if not thousands, of people individually who have made this journey as a partner bearable and survivable... yes, I do mean survivable.

It should never be underestimated just how tough it is on the families and friends who are around a patient undergoing treatment. Emotionally and mentally, it can be exhausting and, without taking the time to rest up and recoup, the people on the outside can undoubtedly suffer trauma.

So, who do I acknowledge?

Well, starting with the obvious, it starts with Amber.

She guided me in many ways to understanding the challenges and what her needs were at any particular stage of treatment.

This was as a direct result of the clear and concise information she received from the oncologist, the oncology team and everyone at the frontline who she came into contact with.

The NHS and the private medical centre professionals, including those that are not visible, the pharmacists, the lab technicians and scientists who diligently, behind the scenes, strive for answers, whether it be diagnosing or identifying solutions, it all matters. They matter.

The charities, that not only provide support to patients and families but fund research to reduce the risk of cancer, provide results and extend lives with purpose, also matter.

Friends and family supported me, and they should all be acknowledged.

The little wins on any one day go a long way to coping, and it can be simply by having an encounter with someone you don't know, on the side of a mountain overlooking a Scottish loch, that cuts right through to your soul and the purpose we give to our lives.

Probably acknowledging the importance of being nice is something we could all sometimes do well to try to achieve that little bit better.

In writing about the experience as a partner in a cancer situation, I do believe that the lessons learnt could just as easily be applied when dealing with any life-changing event.

And finally... I want to acknowledge the courage we all have to face our fears and overcome adversity. In itself, it is something that epitomises the strength of the human spirit.

Love life.

Printed in Great Britain
by Amazon